THE 7 A.M. WORKOUT EDGE

THE 7 A.M. WORKOUT EDGE

WAKE UP, WORK OUT, OWN THE DAY

ANTHONY ARVANITAKIS

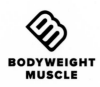

BODYWEIGHT MUSCLE

Hardcover ISBN: 978-1-5445-4104-4

Paperback ISBN: 978-1-5445-4103-7

Ebook ISBN: 978-1-5445-4102-0

To Stavroula.
Your unquestionable faith in me
always helps me stay on my path.

CONTENTS

PREFACE

I DON'T KNOW WHY YOU DECIDED TO READ THIS BOOK.

Maybe it's because you once tried working out in the mornings for a while, and it felt great, but…you just couldn't stick to it.

Maybe it's because you've never managed to stick to an afternoon workout routine.

Maybe it's because even though you feel like you're not a morning person, you are still intrigued to see if you could turn into one.

Maybe it's because you've always felt you wanted something more from your exercise routine than just looking good in a bathing suit.

Maybe you're caught in a slump.

Maybe you feel blocked creatively.

Maybe you're going through a stressful period and looking for a way to deal with all the pressure.

Maybe it's a combination of some or all the above…

What I can tell you is that the 7 A.M. Workout Edge has worked for people in all of these scenarios.

Introduction

March of 2008. It's a little bit after midnight as I'm driving through a dark alley, in a hurry to deliver my final pizza. I suddenly sense a vehicle coming from my left with great speed. I turn my head toward the car, a set of big bright lights blinds me, and… BAM!

I start floating through thin air.

Just like in a typical movie scene, time slows down. What is probably not more than a three- or four-second flight feels like fifteen seconds. As I'm lost in an oddly pleasant state of weightlessness, I hit the pavement. I'm seventy feet away from the crash point (as they inform me later on).

I still haven't understood the severity of my situation. I think of getting up, but I notice that something is wrong with my left leg. When I get a good look at it, I see that the lower half below my knee is twisted, and my ankle… Wait a moment—that can't be right. I close and re-open my eyes to confirm what I just saw. My leg is twisted in a way that (sorry for the graphic image) has left my ankle lying on top of my knee.

"That's probably not a good thing," I tell myself.

It's Like Starting Your Day with an Unfair Advantage

What followed after that night was a long journey of endless surgeries and a lot of physical and mental struggle. Yet, even after everything, I discovered that if you really want it, even missing a leg isn't enough of an excuse to not get in great shape! So, on my quest to learn to stand on my feet again (well—my foot and a prosthetic leg) and figure out the best strategies to create a long-term sustainable workout routine, the 7 A.M. Workout Edge was born.

How we start our morning has a profound impact on how the rest of our day can unfold.

We might think those first fifteen minutes of snoozing and swiping our index finger down on our phone's screen isn't a big deal. But we're not realizing that we're priming our brain for similar behavior patterns during the rest of the day.

It's also important to realize that our cognitive resources are not unlimited, and—like an old computer's RAM—they only fully replenish once we restart our brain the next day after a good night's sleep. When we start our day browsing through social media, we're already wasting brain power to process useless information that has no positive impact on our life whatsoever. Plus, more and more evidence is emerging each day about the rest of the potential negative psychosocial impact social media might have on us.

Next, we might think that starting our day sitting in the kitchen, only to leave our home, sit in our car, and sit again in our office chair should help us feel less fatigued. But then why do we feel so tired all the time? Well, it turns out that spending so much time sitting, aside from not being beneficial for our physical health, isn't doing great things for our mental performance, our motivation, or our energy levels.

Being inactive for long bouts of time during the day often makes our brain think we're getting ready for a nap, so it starts sending melatonin to our sleep center, making us feel drowsy. But then the phone rings or our boss enters our office. Our body responds by sending cortisol and adrenaline our way, and our eyes are wide open again.

Still, this jolt of energy is only temporary. Soon enough, our eyelids start to feel heavy once again. So, we resort to drinking more coffee or energy drinks, pinching our thigh under the desk, or whatever it is we do to push through the day.

Sound familiar?

Here's the biggest problem with all this: feeling sleepy doesn't mean we are actually tired, even though we tend to confuse the two. This is why, after struggling to stay awake all day, we go home and expect to fall asleep right away but often find ourselves in bed with our eyes once again wide open. Annoying, right? It's like our body is messing with us all day in order to torment us even more at night. After a night of poor-quality sleep, we wake up even more tired the next day. And the cycle continues…

The reality is that sitting might feel relaxing in the moment, but too much of it just makes us more tired in the long run. And, of course, there are the rest of the negative physiological impacts it has on our general health. As they say, sitting is becoming the new smoking—and that's based on some pretty valid points.

For example, during prolonged sitting, electrical activity in our muscles drops; and so does the rate at which we burn calories. After three hours, our artery dilation decreases, making blood flow a lot slower. This might not happen to such a huge extent that it's causing us harm in the moment, but the effect compounds dramatically over time. There's even research showing that excessive sitting might increase the odds of premature death.

Life before the 7 A.M. Workout Edge

Here's how a typical day of mine started, about a year before I began taking advantage of the 7 A.M. Workout Edge in my life.

STEP #1

I wake up at 7 a.m. to the worst invention ever created by humankind: the alarm clock. No matter how many times I try to change my phone's alarm-clock tune to something smoother, it still makes the most annoying sound in the universe. I'm being a bit dramatic here, but you know how some mornings can be. I'm exhausted, so I hit the snooze button at least once before I even consider starting to wake up. As usual, I think sneaking in a few extra minutes of sleep might help. But, I wake up again after ten minutes feeling equally tired, if not worse. They say that insanity is doing the same thing over and over again and expecting different results. Yet, I still hit the snooze button each morning expecting to feel better afterward…

STEP #2

I turn on the Wi-Fi on my phone and start scrolling, justifying this activity as professional time I need to spend on my company's social media, even though that's not the only thing I'm looking at. Before I know it, thirty minutes of my morning are already gone, triggering a domino effect of procrastination and chaotic behavior that will carry through the rest of the day.

STEP #3

I force myself to take a look at my appointments on Google calendar in order to snap out of my pointless procrastination. This triggers my anxiety levels enough that I get up and start getting dressed while gulping down a cup of coffee. After that, I'm looking for my keys while trying to pack my backpack in a hasty and inefficient manner.

STEP #4

Around 8:15 a.m., I'm rushing out the door, trying to be on time for my first coaching session of the day. Often, I find myself driving stressed—which is also when I do my worst driving. I barely arrive on time for my appointment. By the way, the plan was also to somehow work out before my appointment, but I tell myself I'll be more organized tomorrow. My client arrives a few minutes after me, and I pretend as if I've been there early enough to be all prepared and look organized and professional. Meanwhile, the sweat on my forehead from trying to quickly and stressfully set up everything is probably betraying my act.

At the end of the day, although I work an average of twelve hours, I always feel I have very little to show for all that time…

Life after the 7 A.M. Workout Edge

Here's a typical day of mine a year later, after having incorporated the 7 A.M. Workout Edge in my life.

I wake up at 6:45 a.m., effortlessly and on most days feeling completely rested. Within twenty minutes I've begun my morning workout. At 8 a.m. I'm out the door, showered and energized. Next, I'm listening to my favorite morning playlist on Spotify, as I'm enjoying a calm drive to work. I'm there fifteen minutes earlier, which gives me plenty of time to set up everything with ease and welcome my first client.

The rest of the day also goes by a lot smoother. Even though I have the same workload I had prior to the 7 A.M. Workout Edge, I finish work one to two hours earlier since I'm a lot more focused and productive, and a lot less stressed. I drink half as much coffee as I used to—which is still plenty, considering I used to drink five or six double espressos per day! But hey, what can I do? I love my coffee; it's one of the few vices I still have! I also don't resort to energy drinks anymore because I simply don't need them. And finally, I feel a lot more rested, even though quantity-wise, I sleep the same seven hours I used to. Quality-wise, though, things are (as you can imagine) a lot different.

Contrary to the past, I feel that *I* set the pace of each of my days—not life or work. Sure, there are days when things don't always run smoothly, and there are days when I lose my mojo, but these are the exceptions. I find myself singing more on my way to work and coming back home after a long day without being pissed off and frustrated—a typical scenario in the past!

I even have time for a personal hobby, something my past-self wouldn't even have considered (I'm learning to play the piano, by the way!). I've stopped obsessing over perfection, and I just focus on doing everything a little better every day. I focus on long-term slow and steady progress over time, not short-term sprints that eventually lead to burnouts and resentment of my job. It's like starting each morning with an unfair advantage and having a head start on the day, which has already begun to feel successful!

This is what the 7 A.M. Workout Edge has done for me. Yes, it can also help you lose fat, build muscle, and get abs if that's important for you as well, but I consider these more as the long-term side-effects the 7 A.M. Workout Edge can offer—not the main benefit or the main driver that keeps you going! By the way, later on we'll be discussing how this mindset leads to even greater and more long-lasting physical results.

What's in It for You?

By reading this book carefully, page by page, you'll gather all the tools you need to become a morning workout person and design a bulletproof personal morning workout routine! I've studied every possible obstacle you might come across, and I've created practical solutions that will help you overcome any problem you encounter—without having to go through the same frustrations I did!

This is not a militant "Just do it!" or *"Get* your butt out of bed, soldier!" type of book. As with any habit, the key is to start small and work with the grain of human nature, not against it!

By taking into consideration how your brain and overall physiology work in the morning, I'll teach you how to create a routine that builds momentum gently—a routine that prepares you both physically and mentally to the point that your morning workout becomes not only as effortless as possible, but also something you look forward to every day, even if you always struggled in the past with getting anything done early in the morning!

In this book, you'll learn basically everything you need to become a successful morning workout person:

- The mental, physical, and other benefits of the 7 A.M. Workout Edge

- Sleep considerations

- How to build and implement an effective routine

- Nutrition

- Addressing challenges and setbacks

Obviously, the 7 A.M. Workout Edge will not fix all your problems, but it can be one of the most potent catalysts for positive change in your life. It can become the lever you need to get unstuck, build momentum, and start making things happen for you again!

As you stick to your morning routine and workout, you'll begin to notice how each successful session becomes a confirmation that your problems do not define you. A punch to the ribs of your doubts, fears, and your inner critic that are holding you back from creating the life you want. It will propel you forward and keep you true to the rest of your goals whenever you feel you're struggling to maintain momentum.

This is the impact your new habit can have on you, and once you experience it, you won't want to miss out on it ever again. Once you learn how to tame your mornings, the 7 A.M. Workout Edge will become your personal secret superpower!

No, the whole process is not going to be a picnic. Especially in the beginning. Sure, I'd like to tell you that reading this book will magically transform you into a morning workout person. But, if you want to build a new habit that has the potential to have a real, positive impact on your life, you have to be invested in it. You have to be ready to put in the work and feel uncomfortable for a couple of mornings.

If you are serious about it and follow through with all the guidelines in this book, you'll be amazed by the effect the 7 A.M. Workout Edge can have on you! Once we get your morning routine perfectly dialed in, you'll begin to see there's something special about training at the beginning of the day while most people around you are sleeping and the town is still peaceful.

Why Did I Write This Book?

After growing a few gray hairs and approaching four decades of being alive on this spinning rock, if I can say one thing with certainty, it's that no matter how many times you'll feel like you've figured things out, life will always find a way to knock you down again. This is a universal law, and the only thing you can really do about it is remind yourself to stay humble and, as cliché as it may sound, learn to get up faster.

What does all this have to do with morning exercise? Well, one of the best ways I've found to get up faster is the 7 A.M. Workout Edge! If you practice everything you learn in this book, you'll realize that if you can manage to get up early and work out on a crappy day, there aren't a lot of other things you can't convince yourself to do after that.

Morning exercise has helped me turn things around during a lot of challenging times. I believe that a morning workout almost has magical powers! It can change how you think, feel, and operate across the rest of the day. Yet, at first, even after seeing the huge positive impact it had on me, I still went through periods during which I struggled to stick to my morning workout routine.

Then I realized the reason why this was happening.

I didn't have a systematic approach! A standard routine that could stand against any turbulence I'd be dealing with! After falling off the morning workout wagon a couple of times, I knew I needed a clear method to help me stay on track every time life decided to throw me a curveball.

I also needed strategies to make sure I didn't go through that classic downward spiral you experience with any habit after missing just one freaking session—even though you've been consistent with your routine for weeks! I was lacking practical steps that would help me with things such as overriding the lazy part of my brain when it tried to make me sleep in. Something had to motivate me, even during those cold winter mornings when I felt tired, and my bed was just too warm and cozy to leave!

Honestly, that was the main reason I stuck to writing this book.

I'd like to sound more altruistic and tell you I did it in order to share all this knowledge with the rest of the world. But, even though I thought that's why I began writing this book, eventually I realized it was also something I did for my own benefit.

This book became a way for me to gather and organize all the information I needed in order to create the perfect morning workout guide.

A manuscript with a pretty cover that could sit in my library, facing me and reminding me what an important role the 7 A.M. Workout Edge has played in my life.

A roadmap I could pick up anytime I needed help to stay on track the moment tough situations arose and started weighing me down or stirred me away from my morning routine.

A big post-it, reminding me of the powerful tool I have at my disposal!

What Do You Have to Lose?

In summary, this book is about incorporating a habit at the beginning of your day that will energize you, improve your mood, and make you more productive and less reactive—a habit that will improve your sleep, decrease your stress levels, and increase the overall quality of your life! It's about creating a new habit that is realistic but enjoyable. Because once you enjoy working out, getting in good shape is just a matter of time!

All it really takes is investing a few weeks to get organized and restructure your mornings. Take all those minutes you spend snoozing, scrolling on social media, reading stressful headlines, or sleeping in after binge-watching episodes on Netflix the previous night… Instead of letting them fall through the cracks of wasted time, we will be reinvesting them in a habit that can have a positive impact not only on the rest of your day, but also on *the rest of your life.*

What do you have to lose other than a few hours of carefully studying this book, and less than half an hour at the beginning of your day testing it out? Assuming we're talking about a habit that can have such a huge positive impact on your life, I think it's a very small cost to pay!

Imagine the Following

Imagine waking up in a good mood and getting your morning workout in as if it is something you've been doing all your life. Instead of feeling groggy as you're leaving home to go to work, you're walking out the door with a smile on your face and a spring in your step.

You arrive at the office in a state of euphoria, with your mind laser-focused and your eyes wide-open. Instead of yawning over a cup of coffee in the morning and gulping down energy drinks to get through the afternoon, you're actually consuming less caffeine than usual, and you can't remember the last time your energy levels were so steady across the day.

Once you're done with work in the afternoon, you can decompress and finish off the day as you please. Instead of having to go to the gym, you can go straight home, have a nice warm shower, wear some comfortable clothes, enjoy a nice home-cooked meal, spend quality time with your family, and read a book. Or, you can have some time for a personal hobby like playing the drums or piano. You can also catch a nice movie with a friend or your significant other.

And finally, imagine yourself at the end of the day effortlessly falling into deep sleep until the next morning.

That's the fastest way I can describe what the 7 A.M. Workout Edge feels like.

So, if all that sounds interesting, keep reading!

PART 1

CAN EVERYONE BECOME A MORNING (WORKOUT) PERSON

INTRODUCTION

It's around noon, and after looking out the window for a couple of hours at snowy Amsterdam from my hospital bed, a nurse enters the room with a smile and tells me in a soft tone that it's time. As I lay on the surgical table, I say to myself, "Well, I guess this is it..." My hands feel a bit shaky as I realize that a part of me will be lost forever. The anesthetic slowly starts to kick in, and my vision becomes blurry. I can only see the gloomy white lights on the ceiling. I start relaxing and enjoying the feeling of weightlessness as I fall asleep...

Rehab after the amputation took close to six months. So, in the beginning of the Dutch summer, I was finally able to confidently walk without crutches again. Every day, I woke up early in the morning and went for a stroll to practice my gait. I loved those morning walks! The feeling of freedom and independence of just being able to walk with no means of support was invigorating! I had gotten rid of the crutches, the canes, and the hunched and depressed posture I had been carrying all those years. I finally began walking with my chin up again.

My whole morning walking routine empowered me to continue the rest of the day with a positive attitude!

But, about another six months later, life got in the way, and I forgot about my morning routine. It took me a few more years to realize how some habits can create a domino effect of positive change throughout the rest of our day when placed strategically early in the morning. Some habits can even become the foundation you can step up on, giving you the confidence to see that more and even bigger achievements during the rest of the day are within your reach!

Morning exercise is undoubtedly one of those habits (if not the most powerful one!). It can give you the mental boost you need to improve your nutrition, cut smoking, and spend less money on pointless things that don't make you any happier; make you better at your job; and the list goes on. Basically, once morning exercise becomes a fixed daily habit, anything else you want to change in your life becomes easier.

Your exercise routine doesn't even have to be anything extreme. Sometimes, even a simple morning power-walk can suffice when you're getting started!

CHAPTER 1

WHAT DOESN'T KILL YOU CAN HELP YOU BUILD BETTER HABITS!

"Rock bottom became the solid foundation on which I rebuilt my life."
—J.K. ROWLING

WE ALL EXPERIENCE A BIG LOSS AT SOME POINT IN LIFE. IT CAN BE LOSING someone in love or losing a loved one—and, eventually, we go through both. Losing a limb is not so different. As a matter of fact, when you lose a limb, you even go through the typical five stages of grief: denial, anger, bargaining, depression, and finally, acceptance.

The worst thing about my accident was that I was left with a leg that was somewhere in the middle of being worth saving and needing amputation. At first, my doctors told me it was worth trying to save but would need about a year and a few more operations. That course of action sounded extremely challenging, since I was only twenty-three years old and the type of person who was highly athletic and not able to stand still for five minutes. Nonetheless, I said okay. At that point, I couldn't even imagine a life without a left leg.

That one year turned into two and a half years and a dispute with my doctors in Greece that made me leave the country to try my luck in Northern Europe. After a few more operations and *another* two and a half years in the Netherlands, all hope was lost. My doctors and I decided it was time, so my amputation was planned for six months later. After a total of five mostly bedridden years and thirteen operations, my final surgery took place on January 17, 2013, at the AMC hospital in Amsterdam.

At that point, I was actually looking forward to my final surgery; getting a prosthetic leg would finally set me free and allow me to get my life back. After fifty-eight months with multiple periods of feeling borderline depressed, intertwined with periods of drinking, smoking, and occasionally other substance abuse, I decided to say "enough" and take charge of my life.

In the end, as painful as it may be, we all know that loss carries the potential for growth. It can make us wiser, kinder, more appreciative, more empathetic, and more humble. So, in the big picture of things, losing a limb and all of those challenging years made me a better and stronger person indeed.

Still, even though this whole "what doesn't kill you makes you stronger" mental framing of our struggles can be true, and even though losses and health scares like these remind us to be thankful for the little things in life, it is almost impossible to maintain this mindset over time. Eventually, it is human nature to simply forget and take everything for granted again.

Instead, what I've found works better is using our hardships to inspire ourselves to change by creating new habits and routines that help us make the best out of life!

Life Gets in the Way

The biggest problem with positive habits and routines is that even if we manage to stick to them for enough time to experience their benefits, we still often fail to keep up with them in the long run. No matter how excited, inspired, and motivated we start out, more often than not, life figures out how to get in the way—sometimes to the point that even our own health and the habits that support it (exercise, nutrition, sleep, etc.) are no longer a priority.

Having coached hundreds of people from all over the world during the last decade, I find that this happens in two main ways:

THE UNEXPECTED, SMACK-IN-THE-FACE WAY

Quickly said, something bad happens, you experience some kind of loss, and you let go. Common examples can typically be a rough break-up, a divorce, getting fired, or losing someone close to you. Or, maybe a huge Jeep crashes into you while you're delivering your last pizza during your side-job as a student (yes, I got a bit more personal in this last example).

THE MORE SUBTLE WAY

After turning into an adult, life slowly becomes busier and busier and a bit more stressful with each year that goes by. Responsibilities keep piling up, workload increases, maybe you start a family, maybe you start a business (maybe both). More people depend on you, and eventually, finding time to exercise while sparing that extra willpower required to eat healthy on a daily basis seems like an impossible task for any average adult in your shoes.

After all, you have to take care of so many more important things other than yourself, right?

I Get It

After my amputation, I told myself that I'd never complain about anything again as long as I was otherwise healthy. But guess what? I still have days when I complain about the stupidest things. And even though I got over the loss of a leg, using exercise as one of the cornerstone habits to lift myself by my own bootstraps, I've still fallen into the trap of neglecting my own health and fitness over and over again!

After all, I'm still human, and that means that every now and then life still finds a way to wear me down or even give me a new, unexpected smack in the face!

Yet, although I'm now thirty-seven years old (as of this writing), and I have a job that takes twelve hours out of my day on average, and I also have a prosthesis that often causes an array of problems I can't always predict, I'm in the best shape of my life! No, I'm not saying this to brag. And no, I'm not in any case the type of person who finds it easy to be militant with his exercise routine and nutritional habits all the time.

Just like everyone, once in a while I'll still lose motivation, I'll still skip a workout, and I'll binge-eat. One of the things I've realized, though, is that in the end, we also have to see fitness a bit like dancing. We all miss a step. The secret is to take it lightly, make it part of the dance, and keep moving.

The reason I'm sharing this is because I used to think that in order to inspire others as a trainer I had to be a role-model and present a flawless image. I had to make it look as if self-discipline was indeed second nature.

That was until I realized that sharing my struggles made me more relatable and inspiring to everyone I wanted to help. So even though I've gotten over the loss of a limb, I don't mind telling you that I've still struggled again with everything else regular life has thrown at me. From a quarter-life crisis, to break-ups, to financial challenges, and all of the other common hits life throws at us.

So, no matter what you're going through, I want to tell you that I get it!

In one way or another, I've been exactly where you are at some point—because, guess what? Even though we might live in different places, speak different languages (I'm Greek, by the way), have different skin colors or preferences, and even though we don't have the same number of toes: we all go through the same emotions and inner struggles.

It's the human experience called life!

Still, with every fall, I've now found that I can use my morning routine to pick me up again. I've discovered the power of morning exercise, and how it can be the first and most powerful step at the beginning of the day while getting through life's challenges. When I felt horrible after a break-up, I knew that all I had to do was get my morning workout in, and the rest of the day would be brighter. When out of the blue a big financial problem knocked on my door, I knew that as long as I trained and didn't snooze in the morning, I'd be less stressed and less mentally paralyzed, and more proactive about figuring things out. And when I got the blues and thoughts such as, "What have I done with my life?" were spinning around in my head in my mid-thirties, my morning routine helped me set new goals and aspirations again.

Whenever something has weighed me down during the last few years, I've always known that everything would be better and clearer after my next morning workout.

CHAPTER 2

CAN EVERYONE BECOME A MORNING (WORKOUT) PERSON?

"An army that cannot yield will be defeated. A tree that cannot bend will crack in the wind. The hard and stiff will be broken; the soft and supple will prevail."
—LAO TZU

THERE'S A NOTION THAT SOME OF US ARE BORN MORNING PEOPLE, AND SOME are not. Sure, some people might struggle a bit more with being functional at the beginning of their day. But, the reality is that any one of us can adopt a morning workout routine once it's set up right.

Sure, I can brag about how effortless getting up in the morning and working out is for me, or how I never make excuses because I've set my mind to it and I'm simply awesome like that, but none of it would be true. Neither is yelling motivational quotes and using brute force to command people to take their lives in their own hands, even though it might make a cool video or post on social media.

When did any of that ever help you create a long-lasting change in your life?

I'll repeat this simply because it's essential to keep in mind when creating your own morning routine: when it comes to habit formation, the key is working with the grain of human nature, not against it!

That is why I'll teach you how to create a morning routine that builds momentum gently and takes into consideration how our brain and our overall physiology work in the morning.

Why Training Like a Movie Star Doesn't Work

After I had my final surgery and got on the road to recovery, I had a year to focus on rehabilitation. No job, no kids—basically, no responsibilities! I had all the time in the world, so I also decided to focus on getting back in shape, both physically and mentally. I started designing my own workout routines; on average, I trained three times a week for about an hour and a half per session. The rest of the day was mostly spent meditating, reading books, cooking, and what I enjoyed most: long walks in the woods!

Just being able to walk again with no means of support was a huge deal after I had spent more than five years being either in bed or on crutches. It was enough to make my whole day! Even nowadays, it's one of my go-to habits to calm down and boost my mood.

Although I spent a lot of time alone that year, it was probably one of the best years of my life! I was happy to be alive, move, walk, and rebuild myself from the ground up. But one day, my rehab was over, and it was time to get back to reality. I started working, and my days shrunk really fast. It turns out that having an office job that requires you to be there for close to ten hours per day while commuting for another two doesn't leave a lot of time for anything else.

At first, I tried to make it work and stick to my ninety-minute workout routine. I told myself things like, "It's just about setting your priorities right," and "I won't make excuses like everyone else." At first, I tried working out after work, which meant that I had to train around 8 p.m., after a long day at work and over an hour of commute on the way back. Soon enough, I realized that I had zero motivation for it.

Next, I tried working out in the morning, which meant I had to be up around 5 a.m. Although it felt brutal, and although I was already not getting enough sleep, I managed to push through it for at least a while. After all, movie stars like The Rock and Mark Wahlberg were doing it—so why not me, as well?

This made things worse. A year later, I ended up stressed and tired with zero willpower left. The sleep deficit made me cranky at first. Later on, it led to weeks of feeling border-line depressed. Eventually, I had my first mental burnout, which took me two months to recover from. But that's what our culture teaches us today, right? At least that's what it did back then. When the going gets tough, the tough get going. Just push harder, work more, sleep less, and don't be such a wuss!

I don't think it's a coincidence that depression and burn-outs were at their peak in the wealthiest and most developed countries where this mentality of "more more more" had become the norm. In the end, the more we have and do, the more we feel we need to keep on doing!

As the popular quote says, we get obsessed with "buying things we don't need to impress people we don't like." Or, as I see it (and to paraphrase the previous quote a bit in order to make it more relevant during an age when social media was born): we spend our life buying things we don't need and doing too much—to impress people we don't like or even know!

Lately, though, this has begun to change a bit. A lot of us are beginning to realize that this way of living is not sustainable and doesn't make us happy in the long run. Don't get me wrong—I like hard work, setting goals, and stepping out of my comfort zone in order to evolve as a person. And sure, sometimes it requires hustling and grinding!

But these times should always be seen as a short-term strategy, fueled by meaningful purpose—and, most importantly, followed by the analogous time required for your body and mind to recover and regain balance. Just like with exercise, you can have peak periods during which you push the pedal to the metal in order to break through plateaus and achieve a special goal. But you also need to allow your body to recover properly afterwards.

Hustling and grinding shouldn't be glorified as a way of living! Sure, it sounds cool when some of your favorite celebrities promote it, but let's be honest: most normal human beings, like you and me, have to be at work early in the morning, don't have personal chefs or trainers, are still trying to establish a business or build a career, and are taking care of a family. So overall, for regular people with a ton of adult responsibilities, waking up at 4 a.m. and working out for two hours is something that is only going to wreck you in the long run!

The All-Or-Nothing Mindset

An all-or-nothing mindset only leads to extremes. For example, when it comes to fitness, people often either train themselves into the ground or go the opposite route and end up completely neglecting themselves. Plus, more often than not, the first scenario leads to the second one. Trying to do too much leaves you overtrained and overwhelmed, thinking there's no other way. So, eventually you just let go.

This is why this is not a book about waking up at 4 a.m., having slept for only four or five hours, and training as if you're the underdog in a boxing movie. I admit I'm a sucker for seventies workout montage scenes and movies where the protagonist wakes up before dawn, drinks up a couple of raw eggs, and starts running around town while shadow boxing. But unless you're training to beat another country's boxing champion, there's no reason to go to such extremes every morning.

Sure, it might look cool and inspiring, but for most people in the real world, it's just a recipe for failure. I know this because I've tried it, and I've crashed mentally and physically by trying to stick to it. It's one of the reasons I changed my mindset and created the 7 A.M. Workout Edge. Movie stars train like action heroes because it's their job. But guess what? You don't have to do the same to be fit, healthy, or happy. Your workout routine should make you feel better during the rest of the day and week, not worse! It should lead to well-being—not burnouts!

It took me years for this mindset to set in, but more complexity is not the answer to dealing with an already complex life. It's common in our times to believe the path to success is paved by working relentlessly; that we have to overthink everything and always overexert ourselves; and that if we aren't perpetually exhausted, we're not doing enough. But sometimes, instead of pushing ourselves harder, it's simply smarter to look for an easier path.

One of my favorite books, *Effortless,* by Greg McKeown, has a very simple rule regarding rest and recovery: "Do not do more today than you can completely recover from by tomorrow." Although this would probably never be the tagline for a Nike advertisement, it's actually a mindset that produces better results in the long run, whether we're talking about fitness or any kind of goal. Sustained effort and consistency over a long time always beats the short-term grinding approach that leads to fatigue and eventually adds up to longer periods of inertia.

However, that long-term mindset has to be cultivated, and it won't sound appealing when you're all fired up to achieve. For a lot of us, it's not something we can understand until we have our first breakdown. I had to go through my own fair share of defeats and fracturing my ego (in addition to my tibia and fibula) multiple times before I started to mature enough to truly grasp this mindset. Eventually, I realized the simple reality that if you're constantly exhausted, maybe the answer isn't doing more and sleeping less.

Maybe it's better to start figuring out ways to get a bit more sleep while simplifying things so you can work a little less. Maybe there's a smarter and more focused way to navigate through life that can lead to better results in the long run—whether we're talking fitness or anything else! Exhaustion is not a prerequisite if you want to be fit, be healthy, and look good.

CHAPTER 3

THE BENEFITS OF THE 7 A.M. WORKOUT EDGE

"Physical fitness is not only one of the most important keys to a healthy body; it is the basis of dynamic and creative intellectual activity."
—JOHN F. KENNEDY

WHEN WE EXERCISE, THOUSANDS OF COMPLEX CHANGES TAKE PLACE INSIDE our bodies. Our lungs bring in more oxygen that travels through the extra blood our hearts pump to our brain, muscles, and the rest of our body, improving the function of all our vital organs. Hormones and neurotransmitters are also telling the body to convert fat into glucose, reduce pain levels, and improve mood, creativity, memory, and overall cognitive function.

In the long run, exercise can have a positive impact on all kinds of physical and mental health markers and problems, whether we're talking about heart disease, blood pressure, obesity, helping us to fend off depression and anxiety, or preventing type two diabetes and autoimmune diseases such as cancer, premature death, and more!

Even simple, plain, good old walking for a few minutes is enough to trigger a lot of these benefits!

Here's what Annabel Streets says in her book *52 Ways to Walk*:

> A twelve-minute walk alters 522 metabolites in our blood—molecules that affect the beating of our heart, the breath in our lungs, the neurons in our brain. When we walk, oxygen rushes through us, affecting our vital organs, our memory, creativity, mood, and our capacity to think. Walking causes hundreds of muscles, joints, bones, and tendons to move in an elaborate, effortless sequence, propelling us forward but also triggering a multitude of molecular pathways, expanding our heart, strengthening our muscles, smoothing the lining of our arteries, shunting sugar from our blood, and switching our genes on and off in a miraculous process known as epigenetic modification.

And yet, even though we all know about these benefits to some extent, they are usually not a strong enough motive to keep us consistent with an exercise routine. At the end of the day, most of us focus on the effect training has on our external image and consider the physical and mental health effects as simple side benefits.

Aspiring to sculpt an aesthetic physique is not a bad thing, of course. As one of my ancient Greek ancestors, Socrates, said: "It is a shame for a man to grow old without seeing the beauty and strength of which his body is capable." Here's the problem, though: sculpting your physique through exercise and proper nutrition takes a lot of time. It's a long journey, and thinking of exercise and nutrition solely as a means to arrive at this destination leads—in most cases—to impatience and stress. Therefore, more often than not, we end up resenting the journey and quitting!

But we don't have to look at exercise so myopically.

Focus on the Daily Rewards

Here's the thing, whether we like it or not: as human beings, we are much more highly motivated to do something if it produces rewards we can experience today rather than rewards that lie somewhere in the distant future.

This is why the best way to make exercise (or any habit) stick is by learning to focus on the daily physical and mental benefits we can reap from it—not the long-term ones! Sure, we all like getting stronger, faster, fitter, and better-looking but exercise can offer so much more than that (especially morning exercise, as I'll be explaining soon)!

In the end, when you learn to focus on the benefits you can reap from a behavior on a daily basis, it becomes a habit a lot more effortlessly. This is why I want to help you to stop looking at your workouts strictly as something you have to do in order to arrive at a specific destination in the distant future (such as losing a certain amount of weight or achieving a specific percentage of body fat). Instead, I want you to turn your workouts into a morning routine and a habit that amplifies your life on a daily basis!

And by the way, guess what else happens when you learn to do all this? What about all those other long-term external physical results we were talking about previously? Not only do they become a lot easier to achieve, but because you'll be focused on the numerous other benefits we've been talking about, they also appear to happen a lot faster! Suddenly, you look at the mirror one day and your stomach is flatter. Suddenly, an old pair of pants is looser. And suddenly, people start to give you compliments!

Oh, and you'll also probably be a lot healthier and live a lot longer!

Post Morning-Workout Benefits

When you work out in the morning, your body also releases hormones and neurotransmitters such as testosterone, growth hormone, GABA, serotonin, dopamine, endocannabinoids and endorphins. Later on, it also helps to lower stress hormones like cortisol and adrenaline. All this results in a biochemical reaction that

- boosts your mood,

- increases self-confidence,

- increases alertness,

- increases your energy levels,

- sharpens your focus,

- increases creativity,

- and even helps you make better decisions.

You might be thinking, "Doesn't that happen if you work out during any time of the day?" The answer is yes. These scientifically proven benefits apply to training at almost any time of the day.

But, if you train in the afternoon, for example, you only get to experience these benefits for a few hours, since they will taper off once you fall asleep. By training in the morning, especially when our mind is fresh and rejuvenated, these benefits can be amplified and spread over the whole day!

So, not only do you get to start your morning with an improved ability to sort out priorities, block out distractions, and better concentrate on important matters at hand; but you also get to ride that post-workout wave of euphoria and improved cognitive performance for a lot longer—*and* during the hours of the day that matter most! The more you observe and focus on these daily mental benefits, the more addicted you get to all of it.

When you stop obsessing over your long-term destination (i.e., a leaner body, the six-pack, or the chest and biceps), you start enjoying the journey. And, as we already said, when you're enjoying the journey, you arrive at the destination a lot faster and a lot more effortlessly. When you focus on internal change, physical change catches up before you realize it! In the end, looking better becomes the natural side effect of something greater.

Starting each morning with more energy, mental clarity, increased cognitive performance, and all those mood-boosting chemicals doesn't just affect how each of your days turns out. It also affects the rest of your week, month, year, and how the rest of your life unfolds!

The Six-Week Morning Workout Edge Challenge

Words can only go so far in describing the 7 A.M. Workout Edge. Unless you give it an honest try, you'll never really know for yourself. You won't know if I'm just exaggerating to make my book sound cooler or if there's really something to it. Unless you take action, the only thing you'll accomplish by reading this book is wasting a few hours of your life.

So, here's my challenge to you: treat this book as a six-week experiment and see what happens. Why six weeks? Because that's the average time I've observed that people need for their physiology to adapt to a morning routine and the time required before you begin to reap all the benefits we've talked about. Although this timeframe is based on personal observation, I've had others confirm it repetitively (even those who didn't consider themselves "morning people").

No, it's not going to be a picnic. It's going to take some patience and personal work—but nothing great comes easy at first. In the end, if what I've described so far is true, you'll see that it's really just a minor investment of time and effort compared to the overall impact the 7 A.M. Workout Edge can have on the rest of your life!

So, what are you going to do?

PART 2

SETTING UP YOUR MORNING ROUTINE

INTRODUCTION

Now, if creating a consistent morning routine still feels like a huge challenge for some of you, that is okay. It means you are taking this seriously. I'd be more worried if you were overconfident. But, you'll be amazed at what is within your reach from keeping an open mind and focusing on consistent work for a few weeks.

During my first surgery after my accident, there was a moment when I said in my head, "I'm probably never going to be able to run again." This made me panic, since I suddenly realized how I loved breathing in the cold and crisp air while jogging and sprinting on the beautiful highlands in northern Greece where I grew up.

Back to today, though: I can once again out-sprint most men my age up a hill. Still, between these two points of my life, I had to change my mindset; and, most importantly, I had to create and stick to habits that made the change possible.

For something that feels out of our reach to become within our reach, there is always a lot of work to do in the beginning. For a new habit to take hold, to the point that it is almost effortless, we need a period of consistent effort and a willingness to step out of our comfort zones.

This is why, in Part 2, we'll need to scrutinize your current morning routine to get rid of all of your pointless behavioral patterns—and to make room for a new routine with exercise at its epicenter.

In the end, by getting rid of bad and toxic habits, by learning how to manage your morning schedule more efficiently, and by using some other behavioral tricks, you'll be able to rearrange your mornings in such a way that you won't need to wake up more than fifteen minutes earlier than your regular wake-up time to get your morning workout in!

CHAPTER 4

CUSTOMIZING YOUR MORNING WORKOUT EDGE

You don't have to be extreme. Just consistent.
—UNKNOWN

JUST LIKE EVERYBODY'S CALORIC INTAKE IS DIFFERENT, SO IS THE AMOUNT OF sleep we require each night. Although most of us need somewhere between seven and eight hours of sleep per night, the exact amount for each person can often vary depending on our personal genetic predispositions, stress levels, physical activity levels, and our overall lifestyle. Another key here is the importance of q-u-a-l-i-t-y sleep!

You can be in bed for ten hours with your eyelids closed, but that doesn't mean you got quality sleep. If you spend half of your hours in bed spinning, waking up every hour and swiping your index finger down your phone's screen, then you're probably not getting quality sleep.

Based on our evolutionary biology, if you want to optimize your circadian rhythm (the internal clock of the body), you should try to wake up close to sunrise and to start winding down around sunset. In theory, doing this can improve your sleeping patterns and help you feel more rested. Still, if it's not practical for you, don't sweat it! What is most important—and what I want you to primarily focus on—is consistency, since our bodies can adapt and reset their circadian rhythm to the times we sleep and wake up. In other words, like most of our habits, sleep thrives on a regular routine.

So, try to keep the times you go to bed and wake up as consistent as possible. It may prove difficult at first, but it's one of the greatest ways to improve the quality of your sleep, and your quality of life in general.

Figuring Out Your Sleep Intake

In order to get started, you first want to determine how much sleep you need. If you're struggling to figure this out, a simple way to do it is by trying an exercise that is also known as *sleep restriction*. By the way, no napping during the rest of the day is allowed until you complete this exercise.

Here are the steps you want to follow for the next week:

1. Ask yourself what is the minimum amount of sleep you need to feel relatively rested in the morning. For most people, it will be around seven hours.

2. Assuming that it's seven hours for you as well, count seven backwards from the time you want to get up in the morning. Don't overanalyze how much time you also need to fall asleep, or other factors, since we want to start this exercise with a small sleep deficit anyway.

3. Let's say you need to wake up at 6 a.m.; this means that you should be lying in bed at 11 p.m.

4. If you feel tired over the next few days, start adding fifteen-minute intervals to the amount of sleep you're getting. Do this by setting your bedtime earlier and earlier while you keep your wake-up time fixed.

5. Keep doing this until the sleepiness you feel during the day is gone.

Once you've reached this point, you'll have a good idea of how much sleep you need. For most people, it will be between seven and eight hours a night.

Customizing Your Morning Workout Edge

Just to be clear here, you don't have to exercise or wake up at exactly 7 a.m. to reap the benefits of the 7 A.M. Workout Edge. I named this book *The 7 A.M. Workout Edge* for two main reasons. For starters, it was the time I originally began training when I first began writing this book. I also wanted to show readers that you don't have to wake up extremely early or spend too much time on exercise in order to get your morning workout edge.

It's funny when I get some aggressive comments online telling me how this time makes no sense for people that have to start their day a lot earlier. My purpose was obviously never to imply that there's something magical about training at *exactly* seven in the morning and not a minute earlier or later!

The only benefit that training at 7 a.m. might have is that it increases your yearly average exposure to natural morning light, something that can be a plus for your circadian rhythm. But in the end, keep in mind that *The 7 A.M. Workout Edge* is just a title I thought sounded cool, and one that resonated with me during my journey while creating this book.

Hey, if it helps, there are multiple ways you can frame it in your head. You can think of it as "done with my morning workout by 7 a.m." or "already in the shower at 7 a.m. after my morning workout," or "already out the door after my workout at 7 a.m."

But that's not what is important here. What is most important is that you determine y-o-u-r ideal workout time based on your schedule and your sleeping needs. Choose a time that makes practical sense for you in order to make this routine sustainable in the long run.

For example, let's say you were Paul, a personal coaching client of mine who happened to work as a bartender. Paul worked each night until 1 a.m. and went to bed, on average, at 1:30. Paul's ideal amount for sleep each night was seven hours. This means that to take advantage of the 7 A.M. Workout Edge, his workout time each day would be 9 a.m. So, in his case, we could say that I helped Paul set up his 9 A.M. Workout Edge! Sure, that's not one of my most typical clients, but it helps make my point here.

Although there are no rules for what time you should exercise in the morning, there are two rules I recommend you stick to for figuring out your ideal Morning Workout Edge.

Rule #1: Train before Work/Adult Responsibilities

To get started, pick a time that allows you to train before work and all of your typical daily adult responsibilities. This includes taking your kids to school, shopping, dentist appointments, etc. It means anything that can get you sidetracked by getting you stuck in traffic or a business meeting, and anything that will make you push your workout to later in the day until you no longer have the time, energy, or willpower for it.

When you train before all these things, your adult schedule does not dictate your workout schedule anymore. You make sure that you never miss your workout due to external factors. You leave very little room for the unexpected to interfere! And you know how expected the "unexpected" tends to be, especially after the world is awake and eager to get in your way the moment you think you've found some free time to work out!

Rule #2: Keep Your Workout Time Consistent

A fixed time carves a habit deeply into your daily routine. It does not matter if you train at 7 a.m., 5 a.m., or 9 a.m., as long as you keep your workout time consistent. Exercising at the same time of the day, even if we're talking about very short sessions, has been linked with both having a regular routine and getting more overall training volume in the long run!

As seen in one study from the journal of obesity, people who trained at a standard time got more overall exercise in the long run than people with an inconsistent schedule.

It's also worth noting that a large number of these people trained in the morning. Determining a standard time that you work out eliminates one extra new decision every day. When you instead have to reschedule your workout time every day, you give yourself room to negotiate.

If you're not in the best mood, if you're feeling less motivated than usual, if you have a busy day ahead of you which is stressing you out, or whatever the case might be, adding one more decision to your day will only increase the chances of you making an excuse to skip your workout. On the other hand, when your workout time is fixed, it becomes unquestionable. Like brushing your teeth or having a shower, it's just part of what you do each day.

A fixed time helps carve any habit deeply into your daily routine—and, when we're talking about exercise, it's a must!

Finally, working out at a consistent time will also adapt your circadian rhythm to morning exercise and optimize your physiology for you to perform better during that time. Sure, you will feel a bit out of sync when you first switch from training later in the day to training early in the morning. But remember that if you stick to it, eventually it will start to feel a lot more natural!

As we already said, just give it six weeks and make sure you keep your workout time as fixed as possible. I recommend not having a bigger deviation than a maximum of five minutes. Until this new habit forms strong roots, the more strict you are with your workout time, the better!

What about Non-training Days?

When it comes to optimizing sleep but also morning routines, some recommend having a steady wake-up time each day, including on the weekends. Personally, I find it healthy and rejuvenating to have one day of the week when you take a break from your usual routine. For me, this day is usually Sunday. It's my day off from work, my exercise routine, my eating schedule (intermittent fasting), and my alarm clock! I'll have anything I feel like for breakfast, and I'll just enjoy a lazy Sunday morning with my girlfriend.

Of course, this doesn't mean that I wake up at noon. Typically, I'll wake up one to two hours later than usual, since my body is used to waking up early. So, even if I have a wild night, I won't wake up a lot later than my usual time. In other words, having an alarm clock-free day once a week will be okay for most people.

That being said, if you're the type of person who can sleep through a next-door explosion and can keep sleeping unless someone wakes you up, I recommend getting up no later than three hours after your regular daily wake-up time.

The reason you want to avoid oversleeping is that waking up too late on a Sunday can mess up your sleeping schedule the coming night. You'll probably not feel sleepy at your regular time, so you'll stay up late, and waking up and working out the next morning will be a struggle. This is also known as Sunday-night insomnia, which will not only have you dragging your feet the next day, but will also throw you off balance for the rest of the week.

Bonus Tip #1

Exposure to natural light in the morning is one of the best ways to wake up, since it causes our brain to begin pulling back melatonin and triggers a release of cortisol, which stimulates wakefulness. Because having natural light in our bedroom during the time we need it is not an option for everyone (especially during the winter when the first light of the day comes a lot later), I found this tip to be one of the best technological hacks that helped me get started with my morning routine:

I have a smart-lamp turn on ten minutes prior to my alarm clock every morning. It makes waking up feel a lot more easy and natural, reducing sleep inertia to a minimum. The lamp I have also has a sunrise effect, which means that it starts out at a very soft low brightness and then gradually increases for the next ten minutes.

But I use this option only when I sleep alone, or when I have to wake up a bit earlier than usual. Otherwise, I find it a bit aggressive on the eyes, and I don't want to disturb my girlfriend. I typically use the softest option (night-light) which is just enough light to wake me up and allow me to navigate around the bedroom.

You can find a link with all the extra information and gadgets in the final pages of this book.

Bonus Tip #2

The best way I've found to wake up silently, when you don't want to wake the person next to you, is with a smartwatch that has a vibrating alarm. I'm lucky because my significant other falls asleep ten seconds after I turn off my smartphone alarm. But I've found using a smartwatch helpful when I've been a guest at someone else's place and wanted to prep for my morning workout routine without disturbing my hosts.

Disclaimer: something to keep in mind if you're a heavy sleeper is that a vibrating alarm might not be sufficiently effective for waking up on time, especially in the beginning when you're first establishing your new wake-up and workout routines.

Bonus Tip #3

If you have the flexibility, it's also okay to vary your workout time a bit, depending on the seasons, to maximize daylight exposure. For example, assuming it is practical, you can train a bit later in the winter (thirty to sixty minutes) and a bit earlier in the summer. Once again, these are minuscule details and nothing to stress about. I'm just covering them in the book because I often receive questions about them. Personally, I like sticking to a fixed time during the whole year.

Stick to a Schedule

Keep in mind that there is no single ideal wake time for everyone. In a perfect world, we wouldn't have a bedtime, and we would go to sleep when our body just fell asleep by itself. Next, we would wake up naturally after the first light of the day hit our bed and after completing our morning's deep-sleep cycle. Unfortunately, that's not practical for most of us living in modern societies with fixed working schedules and other responsibilities.

Plus, since daylight hours can vary significantly based on geographic location and what season of the year it is, for most people, it would be dysfunctional to have a sleep schedule that strictly follows the day-night cycle, when the rest of our responsibilities start at exactly the same time the whole year long.

In order to adapt to the modern world, the next best thing you can do to optimize your body's internal clock is to have a standard wake-up time, making sure you get quality sleep prior to that. In terms of getting quality sleep, nothing works better than exercising at the beginning of the day. It makes you feel more alert during the most active part of your day, and naturally more tired at the end of your day—priming you to get that quality deep sleep when it's time to go to bed.

Of course, it takes some time for your body to get adjusted to all of this, so remember once again that you need to trust the process and give it time.

CHAPTER 5

MOVE LIKE A CHEF

"Clean your space, clear your mind…"
—UNKNOWN

DO YOU HAVE DAYS WHEN LITTLE MENIAL THINGS SUCH AS LOOKING FOR your keys or wallet feel like they take up half your morning? Or days when you try to start working out in the morning but just getting ready for your session takes most of your time?

We often believe that finding time to work out in the morning is impossible. Yet, what we are not aware of is how much time we waste operating in a dysfunctional and chaotic manner after we wake up. We snooze, procrastinate on our smartphones, look for misplaced stuff, and waste time. Instead, a little bit of order and proactivity could make things a lot easier.

No, hastily stumbling around the house, going back and forth pointlessly and becoming stressed while trying to get ready for work doesn't have to be how each day starts; but it often is! Heck, it's how I started each of my days in the pre-7 A.M. Workout Edge era.

The reality is that most of us, even the most busy, can always find an extra half an hour to train in the morning.

But instead, we let time slip through the cracks of disorder and bad habits. Once in a while we'll try to program everything a bit better, but the problem with our hasty lifestyle is that everything goes back to being organized in an unorganized way. Instead of moving with rhythm, we are stumbling across the house, wasting time and energy without even realizing it—the opposite of how a good chef runs his kitchen!

Okay, if you're wondering "What the frack does a chef have to do with morning exercise?" or if you are concerned you accidentally bought a book about cooking, don't worry! You are still in the right place, and it will all soon make sense.

Mise en Place (MEP)

Chefs can teach us a lot when it comes to efficiency. To the untrained eye, the kitchen looks chaotic: people dashing here and there, pots steaming, pans slamming onto burners, and knives chopping. Yet, good chefs always deliver their dishes warm and cooked to perfection, no matter how packed their restaurant is.

The culinary arts have a special phrase regarding how they maintain such efficiency in the kitchen: mise en place (MEP). At its core, MEP revolves around three central values: preparation, process, and presence. Those words may sound vague and even boring, but, when practiced with purpose, they can become profound.

MEP is a French phrase which, when translated word-for-word, means "to put in place." What it really means, though, is creating a hierarchy and an order in the way we do everything. Distilled to its most basic idea, MEP means to move mindfully while being intentional and respectful of time and the rest of our resources.

Eventually, it can become a way of life and a practical philosophy on making the best use of all available resources and doing each thing a little bit better and easier whenever possible.

Although MEP sounds all French and elegant, the truth is that a lot of us are introduced to this concept at a very young age from the same person in our lives—our mother. Most of us never take it seriously until things start piling up, to the point that we can't get anything done anymore. Well, at least that's how it was in my case.

About a year before writing *The 7 A.M. Workout Edge,* I realized I had come to the point where I was stressing all day long about things of minor importance. These trivialities were creating enough friction to make my life a lot more difficult than it had to be.

In the end, I found that sprinkling a few minutes of MEP here and there made a lot more room for what was important and helped me get rid of a lot of pointless stress. It turns out that when it comes to tidiness and order, some proactivity can make a huge difference! (Yes, mother, you were right. Sorry I wasn't smart enough to listen to you earlier!)

Adopting the MEP philosophy might sound like a hustle at first, but it actually saves you time in the long run. It's a pretty simple idea, but embracing it can change your life dramatically, especially if you are anything like me. Some might think that you are born messy and that doesn't ever change. Believe me, though, when I say it can. I was never the organized type of person either!

If you saw my apartment when I was a university student back in my early twenties, you'd realize that I was the definition of a slob. Have you ever seen one of those TV shows that visit people with messy houses and try to help them get everything back in order? Well, I'd probably have been a worthy guest on such a show back then!

And even though I'd like to tell you I changed a lot after my student years, the reality is that there wasn't a huge improvement then, either. Still, if I could change in my mid-thirties, so can anyone.

So, here are the two central tenets of MEP and how you can apply them to your morning workout routine.

1. CLEAN AS YOU GO

A central precept of MEP is the practice of cleaning as you go—also known as working clean! Keeping things neat and sorted out in a way that creates the least amount of friction when you're trying to get ready in the morning can go a long way. This doesn't mean that everything should look as pretty as a minimalist Instagram account. It simply means committing to optimizing your space in terms of organization and ergonomics so that your interaction with all the items that are part of your morning routine is as efficient as possible.

For example, just as good chefs never leave a dirty kitchen behind them, neither should you leave your workout spot that way. Everything before your eyes should look clear and ready for reuse the next morning. This includes clearing out your backpack, tidying the room/space you trained in, and even organizing your bedroom, kitchen, and any space you spend time in prior to, during, and post-workout.

Make sure your workout equipment is well stored, maintained, and safe, just as a chef would do with all his knives and the rest of his cooking gear. Even if you train at a gym, leave things tidy before you go. You'll feel better, and the gym-owner will not wish you ill will as she or he smiles pretentiously while you're exiting the training establishment.

I know this might sound like more wasted time and effort at first, but in the long run, it makes things a lot more efficient. When you learn to work clean, you slowly become more proactive about stuff such as laying out your training gear and clothes for the next day.

When you make sure you restock the kitchen after you finish your last portion of oatmeal, you don't end up frustrated the next day about not having anything for breakfast. When you make sure you have a clean workout shirt to wear the next day, you don't end up making a whole mess in your closet looking for something in which to train.

In summary, the goal of MEP is to give yourself as little as possible to do the following day. So, when you're already busy with something that will affect you the next day, make sure you take care of it now. In the end, physical order supports mental order and vice versa.

2. SLOW DOWN TO SPEED UP

There's a thing called the planning fallacy, which is a cognitive bias first proposed by Daniel Kahneman and Amos

Tversky in 1979. In simple words, one of our most common human tendencies is to underestimate the amount of time needed to complete a future task. We typically think we can get it done a lot faster than we really can. Even if we have a surplus of time and the best intentions to get something done as quickly and as efficiently as possible, it's in our nature to get caught up in our excitement and end up being late.

Then you also have Murphy's Law, which states that anything that can go wrong will go wrong! I think Murphy is a bit of a drama queen. I still like the quote "Hope for the best but plan for the worst." This is why you want to take into consideration the unexpected (traffic and other transportation delays, weather conditions, etc.) and always schedule your tasks by planning some extra wiggle room!

I especially noticed all this when I first started applying the MEP mindset. The more time the MEP mindset freed up for me, the more I felt I could squeeze extra things into my morning routine. So I left no wiggle room, and the moment there was the slightest interference in my program, I found myself blaming and cursing Mr. Murphy and being stressed by the lack of time I had!

This is a common trap, so be wary of it, and remember that MEP is not about doing as many things as possible. It's about eliminating pointless, excessive, and repetitive action in order to set a pace that is relaxed and efficient. It's about moving mindfully and intentionally, and focusing on what is essential, which also brings us to the next MEP tenet.

3. ELIMINATE THE NON-ESSENTIAL

Life doesn't have to be about always doing more and moving faster. Believe it or not, the more you learn to focus on doing less, and doing what really matters, the more successful and happy you become. And there's no better place to start applying this mindset than your morning routine! This is why every action, every tool, and every habit of your morning routine should have a clear purpose. Be honest with yourself about the time you have, and instead of looking for things to add, first look for things you can eliminate. Instead of trying to constantly cram more and more to-dos into your morning routine, give yourself an extra minute to breathe and look out the window as you enjoy your cup of tea. Or, if you really need to add a new task to your schedule, try to at least first think of what unnecessary task can be removed. Before adding a new positive habit, think of a negative one you can replace it with! In the end, when you make extra room for what is essential, and you move slowly and mindfully, you end up being a lot more efficient and—paradoxically—faster in the long run.

Examples of Putting the MEP Mindset into Practice

After each workout, I place my training equipment (gymnastic rings, mattress, bands, etc.) back in its original place. Next, before hitting the shower, I sort out my backpack and clothes to see what needs washing and what is re-wearable for the next day. For example, underwear and t-shirts will usually go into the washing machine while other items such as socks, sweatpants, gloves, etc., might be okay to be used again the next day. So, I stack them on top of each other and replace the items that went in the washing machine.

Hey, I'm already occupied with my clothes as I'm undressing for my shower, so why spend more willpower and time organizing them tomorrow before my morning workout? Why waste time getting aggravated while walking in circles around my room looking for that t-shirt (which I forgot I already put in for washing the previous day)?

Another of my MEP habits is to recite a little poem before I leave the house (I usually train outdoors) and before putting on my shoes: "keys, wallet, watch, water, phone." Okay, not so much a poem as a set of words I recite like a poem. I'm a forgetful person, and I've made my peace with that. So, every time I leave the house, since there's a big chance I'll forget one of these items that are essential to have with me, I simply rehearse my checklist poem.

Prior to my little poem habit, I would typically do the following: put shoes on, leave the house, go to the car, and then yell, "Damn, I forgot my wallet!" or "Damn, I forgot my car keys!" Sometimes, I can't believe I did this for the first thirty years of my life. Genius, right? Now, instead of getting angry at myself half the time when I leave home, I've made it a habit to repeat my little poem before I tie up my shoes, and I'm good to go.

Since everyone is different, you can make it a fun challenge to look for such personal hacks to include in your morning routine. It's just a matter of simplicity and applying the chef's mindset to everything you do: from preparing your backpack, to how you tidy the kitchen and your bedroom, and all the spaces and items that are part of your morning routine!

The 7 A.M. Time-Tracking Challenge

The following exercise will help you put everything we've learned so far into practice. It will show you that no matter how stuffed you feel your mornings are, you can still declutter and optimize things if you focus on what matters. I like to call this The 7 A.M. Time-Tracking Challenge.

All you need is a notebook or a note-taking app on your phone to log everything you do each morning, from the moment you wake up until the moment your day's main responsibilities begin. Try to be as detailed as possible!

For example:

- 6:30 a.m. alarm clock goes off

- snooze until 6:40

- check social media on smartphone until 7

- get up and visit WC

- make coffee

- etc.

I guarantee you that you'll still observe plenty of pointless behaviors or ways you can better organize your morning. Don't spend too much time on this yet; just make a detailed list of how you spend your time in the morning and look for a few ways you can optimize things based on the MEP principles. Don't worry if you don't have any great ideas yet, either, since I'll be giving you a lot more tips and we'll be taking this to the next level pretty soon. Until then, remember the general mindset of what we've covered so far:

- Act quickly but steadily.

- Pace yourself—but don't waste time, either.

- Be conscious of your actions, but don't overthink everything.

- Move with rhythm, like a chef!

CHAPTER 6

THE 7 A.M. WORKOUT EDGE GOLDEN RULES

"Remember, technology is a great servant, but a terrible master."
—STEPHEN R. COVEY

IF YOU WANT TO BE INTENTIONAL WITH YOUR MORNING ROUTINE, you can't begin your day snoozing or procrastinating on your phone.

In order to maximize the 7 A.M. Workout Edge, you have to set some ground rules, or what I call "The 7 A.M. Workout Edge Golden Rules!" It was only when I began to follow these rules strictly that working out in the mornings began to have a great impact on the rest of my day. After sticking to these rules for a few weeks and sticking to my morning routine, the 7 A.M. Workout Edge took full effect! I saw my anxiety gradually diminish as I started my days with a more positive outlook and I was a lot more clear-headed, focused, and confident!

Rule #1: Don't Snooze

I don't know if you've noticed this, but snoozing rarely helps you wake up better than you did the first time your alarm clock went off. As a matter of fact, it often leaves you feeling lousier. Here's why that happens:

First of all, it's important to understand that sleep is not linear and uniform. Instead, every night you go through several rounds of sleep cycles (four to six of them on average) that can last anywhere from one to two hours. Each cycle consists of four individual stages. Our first three stages of sleep are lighter and are called non-REM (non rapid eye movement).

The first stage is essentially the "dozing off" stage, and it normally lasts just a few minutes. Like when you're watching a TV show before bed and you're starting to drift away. During stage two, our temperature drops, muscles relax, and our heart rate and breathing slow down. This stage can last anywhere between ten and sixty minutes.

Stage three is also known as deep sleep, as the body relaxes even further. This stage is vital for physical recovery (growth and repair of tissues, bones, and muscles) and boosting your immune system.

Our last stage is called REM sleep—and the weird thing here is that brain activity actually increases, reaching levels pretty similar to those that occur when we're awake. Meanwhile, the body experiences temporary paralysis of the muscles, with two exceptions: the eyes, and of course the muscles that control breathing. Even though our eyes are closed, there is rapid movement, which explains the name of this stage.

REM sleep is essential for our cognitive functions (memory, learning, creativity, etc.), and it is when we have our most vivid dreams, which is why brain activity picks up at this stage. In total, REM stages make up around 25 percent of sleep in adults, and getting enough REM sleep is crucial for feeling sharp and focused the next day.

After your alarm clock goes off the first time, your body ends the sleep cycle you're in, and you can either wake up or hit the snooze button and go back to sleep. When you choose to snooze, and your alarm goes off for the second time, you wake up at the beginning of a new sleeping cycle— before you get any helpful, restorative sleep! This is why those extra five to ten minutes of sleep aren't doing you any good; nor do they make it easier to wake up. On the contrary, most times they make you feel foggier and even more disoriented, since you're probably at the end of stage one and haven't had the time to complete a stage of deep sleep that would actually make you feel better.

In a perfect world, we wouldn't need alarm clocks. We'd wake up when our body would naturally come out of its deep sleeping stages, and we'd go on with our day. But, if you're an adult with a job and responsibilities, this approach usually isn't practical. The only way to improve how you feel when your alarm clock goes off is training your circadian rhythm by waking up every day at the same time. This might take a while, but after a few weeks, you'll notice that you'll begin to feel a lot better.

Still, I won't lie to you! No matter what you do, that first minute after your alarm clock goes off won't ever become completely effortless. This is simply something you have to embrace. The way I deal with it is by reminding myself of the bandage example. Here's what I mean: think of waking up like removing a sticky bandage from your forearm or a wax strip from your leg. You can either pull it off quickly, all at once, and start your day; or you can snooze, which is like removing the bandage almost all the way to the end, and then putting it back again—only to try to rip it off again ten minutes later!

If you've been a chronic snoozer, waking up as soon as your alarm goes off will require practice and will be unpleasant at first—especially on days that your alarm clock gets you during the middle of a deep sleep cycle, which feels horrible. But you have to work on it! So remember the bandage example, and I promise things will slowly improve! In the end, getting up the moment your alarm clock goes off becomes a skill. The more you do it, the better you become at it.

Rule #2: Seriously, Do Not Snooze

A few nights ago, I put on a random episode of *Seinfeld* (an old sitcom show). Famous comedian Jerry Seinfeld made a joke during the episode that I thought was both funny and quite true at the same time...

> If any invention marks the decline of human civilization, I think it would have to be the snooze alarm. The snooze alarm is based on the idea that when the alarm goes off, you are not getting up. You're not even awake, you're already a failure. They should sell

the snooze alarm with an unemployment application and a bottle of tequila. Just make it a complete pathetic loser kit!

Yes, rule number two just re-emphasizes rule number one—because you'll probably forget everything you just read the moment your alarm clock goes off again tomorrow morning, even with as much sense as it might make now. Especially if you've been a chronic snoozer, you'll observe how your finger will almost reflexively aim for the snooze button the moment you wake up.

What I consider the biggest problem when it comes to hitting the snooze button has a lot to do with what Jerry mentions. When you hit the snooze button the moment you wake up, you start your morning by failing at your first task of the day! As innocent and as inconsequential as this might seem, by violating the agreement you made with yourself last night about waking up at a specific time, you begin your morning with a failure mentality that builds negative momentum for the rest of the day.

Instead, when you skip the snooze button and put your feet on the floor, you start your day with a small win. This small win gives you a spritz of dopamine, a feel-good brain chemical linked with motivation, and each step after that becomes easier.

Remember, the first step of any habit is the hardest one! Like pedaling a bicycle, it takes more effort to push the pedals in the beginning. Once the bike starts to roll, though, it's relatively easy to maintain momentum. The same is true for the 7 A.M. Workout Edge. So, next time you wake up in the morning dreading the alarm clock sound, fight that impulse to snooze by reminding yourself that getting out of bed is like that first heavy rotation of the bike's wheels. After that, each subsequent choice becomes more and more effortless!

WHAT IS THE BEST ANTI-SNOOZE HACK?

There are alarm clocks that make you solve a puzzle before you can turn them off. I've even heard of alarm clocks in the past that used to donate money to a cause you hated if you pressed snooze. I couldn't find these anymore, though, so I'm thinking someone woke up pissed off and started suing the manufacturer. Overall, there might be many gizmos and anti-snooze hacks you can try out, but I'll save you the hustle, money, and time by sharing the best one.

After researching this topic and reading almost everyone's opinions online, I eventually came back to the classic trick that never fails: leaving your alarm clock in another room.

Nothing really beats that, especially if you're a pathological snoozer! It's way too easy to hit snooze if all you have to do is raise your arm a few inches and hit a button or tap on a screen. Instead, put your alarm out of reach and make sure the volume is loud enough. Yes, this will be annoying for your significant other who might be sleeping next to you, which is why I also offer other tricks later on. But, if you really struggle with snoozing, this is the only way to teach yourself to skip it.

Rule #3: Practice Intermittent Media Fasting

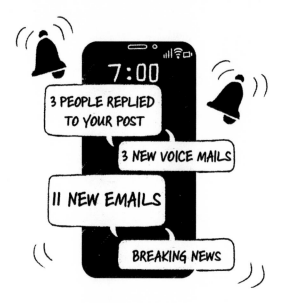

Like it or not, smartphones nowadays have become an extension of our hand. Although they can help us be more productive and improve our life, they can also be a major source of distraction and stress. Just like our mind, our smartphone can be a wonderful servant but a terrible master.

Living in the smartphone era means that we are constantly available to colleagues, our boss, family members (those we like, but also those we don't like so much) and our friends (again, those we are fond of, and those we are not so fond of). All these people are able to hijack our time at any given point.

According to researchers from the University of Texas at Austin, the mere presence of your smartphone can significantly reduce cognitive capacity—even when the device is turned off! More and more research is showing that all this interaction we have with our smartphone increases anxiety levels and decreases mental clarity, especially when we start our day this way.

The best way I've found to keep smartphone use more in the sphere of my control is intermittent media fasting (IMF). IMF controls daily social media intake just as intermittent fasting helps you control your daily calorie intake. For those who are not familiar with Intermittent fasting, it is a popular dietary approach that allows you to consume food during a specific window of time during the day.

Usually, this entails skipping breakfast and not eating anything until around noon, having an eating window between noon and 8 p.m., and fasting again until the next day. Intermittent media fasting (IMF) follows a similar pattern: you start your day by skipping any consumption of digital information, whether that's news, email, or social media.

By abstaining from any media consumption in the morning, we can start and plan our day with greater clarity, and we make more room for creative thinking. We also reserve more brain power and focus for the important tasks that will be coming up next! Lastly, IMF can help us consume media with intent and purpose later on, especially if we turn it into a deliberate activity (additional tips on this soon).

Research shows that most people check their mobile devices the moment they wake up, which is when our brains and our subconscious can be very receptive. In other words, our mind is more prone to passive consumption of information the moment we wake up. I like to equate starting the day with social media with having junk food for breakfast.

When you start your day with a fatty, sugary choice like a donut, your body will just keep on craving things that have the same exciting impact on your taste buds for the rest of the day. This means that a salad and a protein-dense food for lunch becomes a very dull choice. But what about something like nachos and salsa? Now that's such a better follow up, isn't it?

It's the same downhill spiral with media consumption in the morning. The more we feed ourselves with social media and stressful news at the beginning of the day, the more desensitized we'll be when it comes to focusing at work or getting in the mood to read a decent book. Whether we admit it or not, our morning screen-swiping habit is a big waste of time and cognitive resources which we could otherwise invest in more meaningful things and positive habits.

Examples of better things to spend our time on could be our work, creative thinking, real human connection with people we actually care about, investing in educating and improving ourselves, and—lastly—something that just came off the top of my head: how about investing in the 7 A.M. Workout Edge?!

STARTING YOUR DAY WITH SOCIAL MEDIA

Let me ask you a question: would you randomly allow hundreds of people (or more) into your house first thing in the morning, before you'd even opened the curtains to let some light in? People filling your mailbox with requests and advertisements, people complaining and shouting their opinions in your living room, and people spreading out newspapers and articles with the most stressful and often blown-out-of-proportion current news from all around the world on your coffee table?

I'm guessing not.

Yet, that's how a large number of us start the day. Yes, I'm talking about swiping our index finger down our social media feeds and checking our social media inboxes. The moment we tap on that screen and connect to the internet, we are really opening Pandora's box. We're activating a device that is about to bombard us with new messages, emails, to-dos, and other stimuli—all bidding for our attention. What starts out as a quick little check-in often turns into fifteen, twenty, or even thirty minutes or more of our morning being wasted on our smartphones.

We can find all kinds of toxic and pointless behavior on these platforms—and, what's worse, whether we are aware of it or not, is that we're often also part of them. Social media is the perfect place for anyone looking to vent about everything from politics to the next horrible thing that is about to happen. It's also a great place to search for validation through all kinds of unhealthy and pointless ways.

Now, all of this creates a vicious cycle, and before we know it, we find ourselves envying other people's polished, movie-trailer-version lives because our own raw, unedited life can't compare to theirs. If we're having a bad week, we look for excuses to get into a heated discussion and take it out over there! If we're feeling down, we take out our credit card and order something we didn't know we needed until that "random" ad stopped us from scrolling downwards.

Okay, I might be focusing a bit more on the negative side of things here. And yes, there are people out there on social media promoting great ideas, causes that make a positive difference, and all kinds of good stuff. But that's not what your mind will focus on first thing in the morning. When you haven't had the time to wake up properly, your mind will get triggered by things that appeal mainly to your primitive brain. That typically means things that focus on uncertainty, drama, anything that poses a threat to us, and anything that gives us a quick libido high.

For example, one of the most basic primitive instincts social media relies on is making you feel that you're not keeping up with the rest of the "tribe." So, you keep checking what's going on and you keep comparing yourself to everyone else. And while you're trying to present a more polished version of yourself with every post and interaction, subconsciously making sure you won't be ostracized by society, what you're not noticing is how all you're really doing is becoming a slave to your little screen!

And although these platforms seem free, keep in mind that this is not the case. As the saying goes, "If you're not the customer, you're the product being sold." Looking at social media is like having a supercomputer pointed at your brain. When you log in to your favorite social media platform, you're activating computing power worth billions of dollars.

This supercomputer knows what everyone on planet earth with an internet connection likes to click on, and it also has a complete history of our preferences over the years. By observing things such as when we linger on or scroll past a post, it knows what tends to grab our attention. It can predict with great accuracy what content will most resonate with us to keep us in front of our screen just a bit longer so the platforms can keep earning ad revenues!

It also has an armory of psychological techniques based on behavioral science and things such as casino slot machines. Take, for example, the classic *drag down to refresh* gesture. This feature encourages compulsive scrolling by exploiting a phenomenon known as variable rewards. When you can't predict if refreshing the screen will bring you interesting posts to read, the uncertainty makes you more likely to keep trying, again and again—just as you would with a slot machine! Although this may sound extreme to some, it is these exact mechanisms that make social media platforms so addictive!

More and more studies are revealing the negative impact social media use might have on our mental health, linking it to depression, anxiety, low self-confidence, and low self-esteem. It's pretty early to say whether social media affects some or all of us, and to what extent. I believe social media platforms can bring out the worst in us if we let it.

Don't get me wrong; I still think social media can also be helpful if we're extremely intentional and strategic in how we use it. But, with documentaries such as *The Social Dilemma* and a lot of tech experts sounding the alarm on the dangerous human impact of social networking, I'm not sure how much control we'll eventually have (or think we have) over this interactive technology.

EMAIL

In the past, I would constantly get interrupted by email notifications during the day, which would distract me from whatever task I was doing at the time. This started the moment I woke up and kept on going through the rest of the day. At work, I would check email and wonder if I had to reply right away or remain focused on the current task. A lot of times, even if I'd decide to reply later, I'd be doing the task at hand while thinking about the email that messed up my focus, still stressing about how to answer it.

As a result, I would spend double—or even triple—the amount of time doing anything. Especially when it comes to tasks that require heavy focus, a seemingly innocent interruption can cost you a lot more time than you think. Sure, you can just check your email for ten seconds, but getting back to that focused state you were in previously (or, as some call it, "the flow"), might take you another fifteen to twenty minutes! Multiply that by however many times you check your email, or any notification on your phone during the day, and do the math!

The end result? Even though I spent a lot more time on email than I do nowadays (and less time on getting the rest of my tasks done), I also found myself having to spend extra time on email at the end of the week, working past my regular hours to make sure I got through all my messages. This continued until I realized it was so much extra stress and work for no reason!

You see, although answering your email as fast as possible might seem like the best way to keep your inbox clean, it's really just a Pyrrhic victory (a victory that is not worth winning because so much is lost to achieve it). Think about it. Every email you send triggers a response, and that just results in even more incoming emails. Therefore, the more often you reply, the more emails you get. It's a vicious cycle!

Fifteen years ago, technologist Robert Scoble pointed out that for each email he sent, he got 1.75 to two messages in return. This only highlights the unscalable nature of most email productivity systems, and that the only sustainable system to manage email better is answering it less often!

Research shows that monitoring work emails outside of actual work hours negatively affects our mental health and relationship with our significant other. It also shows that checking email less frequently can lead to lower stress levels. Julie Morgenstern, author of the book *Never Check Email in the Morning*, says that "when you check your email or notifications first thing in the morning, you never recover. Those requests and those interruptions and those unexpected surprises and those reminders and problems are endless."

This is why one of the most productive decisions I've made in the last few years is to never check email in the morning. Instead, I only check email once a day, and I do it during working hours. Of course, I didn't manage to do this from one day to the other. At first, I simply started off with postponing my morning email check until I'd be done with my workout. In the beginning, I even uninstalled the Gmail app on my smartphone because I couldn't resist peeking at my inbox before leaving the bed.

After I could manage not checking my email until I was done with training, I postponed checking my inbox until noon. And, once that became easy, I only checked once a day at the end of my working schedule.

Here's my system today for those who might be looking to try it out: although I've reinstalled Gmail on my phone, I don't have email notifications. There's no email so urgent that neglecting it will cause a tragedy. If someone is dealing with a matter of life or death, I don't think he or she will email you. I'm guessing that all the people in your life whom you care about being safe are smart enough to call you or 911.

So, every afternoon, after I'm done with the most important work-related tasks of the day, I set a twenty-minute timer, and I spend that time solely answering email. I start with the messages that are most urgent, and I move my way through the rest. After that, I ignore my inbox until the next afternoon. And that's it!

Although I struggled to apply this rule at first, after seeing how much more productive it's made me, it gradually became a no-brainer. And my inbox has never been tidier! The great thing about this rule is that the more you stay consistent with it, the less time and cognitive resources you end up spending on email. Sure, there are periods when things might get a bit more crammed, but as long as I stick to my twenty-minute rule each day, my inbox never becomes overwhelmingly flooded. It's kind of like keeping your house tidy.

Spending a little bit of time each day to keep it decent usually works a lot better than neglecting everything until the weekend when you have to deal with what looks like a warzone. In the end, the more I stick to the twenty-minute rule per day, the easier it becomes. And a lot of times, I'll be done before my timer goes off!

THE NEWS

We've long known that exposure to the news is linked to negative stress-related emotional responses, as it can increase anxiety, worry, and irrational thinking. Just like social media and email, it's the same vicious cycle, which is why I won't elaborate again on how starting your morning with the news can influence the rest of your day.

I'll just point out one final interesting fact for you to keep in mind: even though only about 50 percent of smartphone users check the news intentionally and on a regular basis with their devices, social media outlets are inextricably tied to the twenty-four-hour news cycle. As a result, a lot of adults under the age of fifty now get their news from social media. Even if you sign into your social media early in the morning without intending to open news apps and websites, you're still getting the news!

No, I'm not telling you not to stay updated with what's happening in the world. But, if you want to fully benefit from your morning workout edge, I definitely advise skipping any form of news until you're done with your morning routine.

Final Tips

Most of us burn a ton of hours on social media, news, and digital inboxes every week—hours that at the end of the year add up to days or even weeks of wasted time. No, I'm not saying to get rid of your phone; and I get it if email, social media, or watching the news is important to you or your line of work. What I do recommend, though, is simply to ignore it all until you're done with your morning workout. After that, feel free to regulate all of it in whatever way makes the most practical sense for you. Personally, I check social media once a day, together with my email check, at the end of my working schedule.

This is not going to be an easy battle to win. In the beginning you'll be at war with your own neurochemistry. Up to now, for most people, the fact is that your brain has been used to receiving a dopamine hit each time you've started your day by checking social media, the news and email, to make sure all is good with the "tribe." As we mentioned earlier, dopamine is a feel-good neurochemical linked with motivation, and it can also give us a feeling of reward.

Our brain has a tendency to get hooked on all these feel-good sensations, the same way an eight-year-old can get hooked on waffles for breakfast. This is why our mind will do whatever it can to make us repeat whatever familiar behaviors will trigger these kinds of neurochemical responses.

So, being intentional with how and when you consume information through your smartphone or other devices is not going to be easy—but it is a game changer once you learn how to do it. And there's no better place to start practicing than in the morning!

I like to see it like this: since replacing a negative habit with a new positive one is one of the best ways to change a behavioral pattern, all you have to do is simply turn your workout routine into your new positive daily distraction with which you'll begin each morning from now on. Don't worry, I'll be providing several more helpful strategies for you to accomplish this. But until then, here are some other easy tips to apply that might help you get started with IMF.

Tip #1: Turn your phone's Wi-Fi and notifications off before you go to sleep, and keep them turned off until you finish your morning workout.

Tip #2: If you want to take more drastic measures, use a classic old-school alarm clock and keep your smartphone out of reach until you're done with your workout.

Tip #3: Lastly, if you need an even more extreme measure, here's something I did in the beginning to help me get unhooked from social media—my biggest struggle when I first started applying the three golden rules.

Having a lot of people follow my work through social media platforms, I had developed this anxiety around answering anyone that needed my help on a daily basis. As you can imagine, it became quite draining after a certain point. So, I uninstalled all my social media on my main smartphone, and I got a cheap second-hand smartphone.

The main prerequisite for this phone was that it could support all of my social media apps—nothing more, and nothing less. It didn't have or need a special camera or any other expensive features. So, if this sounds like an interesting idea to you, keep in mind that it can be a relatively inexpensive smartphone. You can even find one for free by asking a few friends and relatives if they have an old smartphone they're not using any more.

I kept this phone in a kitchen drawer that wasn't easily accessible, and I only used it once a day. The purpose of all this was to make it a bit more of a hassle to access my social media, which otherwise simply required my reaching into my pocket. By creating enough friction between my urge to check my social media and the actions required to act upon this addiction, it became easier to be more conscious of my choices and practice some self-restraint.

Specifically, I only allowed myself to get back to the most important messages within fifteen minutes, every afternoon after work. As extreme as this tip might sound, it helped me to realize that being intentional with my social media usage was possible, and it acted as a stepping stone on my way of getting rid of my social media addiction. I no longer have a second phone, but ever since I did, I've felt that I'm the master of my phone. Very rarely do I slip into a social-media binge.

CHAPTER 7

CONQUERING THE MORNING BATTLE

"Say no to many good things so you can say yes to a few great things."
—GREG MCKEOWN

I'M GUESSING THAT AT LEAST SOME OF THE INFORMATION IN THE BOOK SO FAR is not brand new to you. You've probably heard and read about some of it in other books, websites, health blogs, business-insider types of articles, YouTube videos, or podcasts.

Most of us are aware that swiping away on social media while comparing yourself to other people's photoshopped life or getting riled up by people talking in capital letters and controversial news headlines probably isn't the best way to start your day.

We all know on some level that pushing through each day by overconsuming caffeine and energy drinks that sound as if they're named after a metal band is not a healthy long-term strategy.

Yet, even though we are aware of all of this, we still end up stuck in this cycle of repeating most of these behavioral patterns—not only because we're used to it and it has become convenient, but also because life is hard. Because when you're pressured by time and responsibilities, and you feel like you're carrying the world on your back, there's not a lot of energy for changing such stuff.

Sure, change requires some extra willpower at first. It means stepping out of your comfort zone and walking in an initially unknown territory. But, what if the return on investment is too big to ignore? What if you could hack your brain in the morning in order to turn things around? What if the right dose of exercise at the beginning of the day could help you wake up better, have more energy, and sleep better the coming night? What if you could create a morning routine that felt more like a personal ritual? And what if this new ritual became a new habit you looked forward to every day?

It's all totally possible! And the more you put into this routine, the more you begin to enjoy it—and the positive cycle of its benefits!

No One Is Born a Morning Person

No one, including me, wakes up in the deep winter, while it is still dark and cold, thinking "Awesome! I get to leave my nice warm bed and work out instead of sleeping in for twenty minutes." No, no one is naturally a morning person. We decide to become one, just as we decide to make the best out of our life.

So, what do you do, then? Where do you start after you make the decision to become a morning person? Well, you can try applying the "stop whining and just do it" mindset, which you'll usually hear coming from loud, militant types of personalities. And although these people might be inspiring, especially on social media feeds, that's where their advice usually stays since it rarely has any practical use for the rest of us.

The truth is that motivation is never a good strategy for setting long-term habits because it is based simply on how you feel at a specific moment. I'm not saying that motivation is bad. I actually recommend that you try to cultivate it on a daily basis. As a favorite quote of mine by Zig Ziglar says, "Motivation doesn't last, but neither does bathing; that's why we recommend it daily." What I am saying is that motivation should not be your core strategy because human emotions are unpredictable, and they can change from one moment to the next!

The Big Morning Battle (Lizard Brain versus Prefrontal Cortex)

Those first twenty minutes of the day after our alarm clock goes off are difficult for all of us. And that's not because we're lazy; it's more because of our human physiology. You see, the moment we wake up, there's a big battle going on in our heads that can determine the rest of our day.

This battle occurs between the primal part of your brain (limbic system), which I'll refer to as the lizard brain, and the more recently evolved part, known as the prefrontal cortex.

As you might already know, your lizard brain cares mainly about things that revolve around survival and passing along your genes. Things such as food, shelter, and repro-duction. It has a very short-term perspective, and therefore it will typically direct you towards temporary gratification over long-term balance and happiness.

So, when our alarm clock goes off in the morning while we're in a comfortable bed with a roof over our head and food in our belly from the previous night, our lizard brain won't be particularly motivated to leave this perfectly safe and cozy environment. Unless it gets way too bright in your room and you start feeling extremely hungry, thirsty, or consider your life threatened in some way, your primal brain would rather have you hibernate in this perfect nest.

Another example would be overeating when food is available. Although this would be a good strategy in the past when food scarcity was a common scenario, it doesn't equate to one's well-being anymore. So, the problem with our primal brain's tendencies in today's world is that they usually don't align with what is good for us, and still they tend to drive a lot of our actions!

Our prefrontal cortex, on the other hand, is the more analytical and logical part of the brain. It's the reason we can set goals that can make our lives better in the long run. And the fact that these two parts of our brain are in constant clash is one of the biggest reasons we, the modern man and woman, struggle so much. In the end, the ability to fight our primal impulses and delay gratification is one of the best predictors of success in life and something that we can improve, just like any skill.

Taming Our Groggy Morning Lizard Brain

Now, here is the bad news: when it comes to the lizard brain, daytime blood-flow returns to normal the moment you wake up. This same process takes an extra twenty minutes when it comes to the prefrontal cortex! This is why we naturally gravitate towards comfort and laziness the moment we open our eyes in the morning. It does not mean we are lazy people or not morning types; it simply means we are experiencing the pull of about two hundred thousand years of primal wiring!

This is why we feel groggy during those first twenty minutes. For us coffee drinkers, it's also why we feel we can't get anything serious done without a cup of warm java first, even though that's more of an illusion! Sure, coffee can help, but keep in mind that caffeine can take up to thirty minutes until it has any serious effect on your brain.

The reason you feel more awake the moment you have that first cup of coffee is not so much the coffee itself. Rather, it's the time you spent getting out of bed, putting something on, and making and drinking the coffee! Which, if you count from the moment you leave your bed until you have your first sip, is a process that keeps you typically busy for at least fifteen to twenty minutes.

In other words, your lizard brain is usually the one in charge during those first twenty minutes of the day, while your prefrontal cortex is more like a really old computer that needs twenty minutes to boot properly. The good news, though, is that we are also at a point in our evolution where we can teach ourselves to resist our primal impulses.

What makes us different from animals is that we can tame our lizard brains, even during those early morning hours when the prefrontal cortex is still half asleep. And one of the best ways to accomplish this is by forming routines! Routines program our behavior so we can learn to use our lizard brain, instead of ending up being used by it.

In other words, in order to override the grumpy and groggy part of our morning limbic system and give the prefrontal cortex some time to boot properly, we need to program our brain with a set of simple, clear instructions we can follow as blindly and as effortlessly as possible. This is what I call a "Brain Start-up Routine!"

The Brain Start-Up Routine

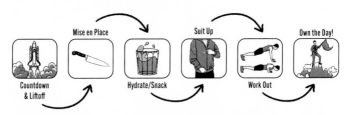

The brain start-up routine (BSR) is also based on an important factor called automaticity. Automaticity is the ability to do things without occupying the mind with the low-level details, allowing us to use an automatic response pattern. This is the result of purposeful repetition and practice, and habits and routines highly depend on it.

This "automaticity" feeling has been described in multiple studies, including systematic reviews in *Health Psychology Review* that analyzed 52 studies. These studies have shown that physical activity can be regulated to a big extent by non-conscious processes such as habits, automatic associations, and priming effects—which is what the BSR is based on!

In other words, your BSR is a set of simple and clear actions that precede your morning workout and help you automate your behavior during the first twenty to thirty minutes after your alarm clock goes off. It is a routine that takes advantage of the automaticity factor and reduces the mental effort and motivation you need in order to reach the point of working out in the morning.

So, to get started, all I want from you is the following: instead of waking up and feeling overwhelmed by the thought that you "have to" work out, from now on, just focus on your BSR!

Take your BSR one step at a time and allow each of these steps to build momentum gradually. This process "warms up" the prefrontal cortex and propels you forward until the point that motivation is no longer critical! Naturally, you'll have to apply more willpower and self-discipline in the beginning; but, gradually, your BSR will reach a level of automaticity that will make it, well, almost automatic.

Even though motivation, willpower, and self-discipline are not means we want to rely on in the long run, you'll have to apply some of them in the beginning until you form a BSR that smoothly primes your brain and body for your morning workout. If you stick to this process and all the guidelines in the book, you will reach a point that your morning routine will begin to feel effortless.

Creating a Custom Brain Start-Up Routine

Each person's BSR, just like each person's personality, will be a bit different. This chapter will show you how to design your own BSR in four steps. These steps are not based on any groundbreaking tactics. Keeping them simple and setting them in the right order is what makes them effective. I recommend that you practice all four of these without any major changes for at least six weeks. After that, feel free to start adapting and refining them in any way you find more practical for you.

Remember, clear instructions and repetition are crucial for lightening the cognitive load of your BSR!

STEP #1: COUNTDOWN (THREE, TWO, ONE... LIFT OFF!)

In her book *The 5 Second Rule* (two million copies sold, Audible #1 Nonfiction Book of the Year, and the sixth Most Read Book of the Year on amazon.com), Mel Robbins explains how to overcome challenges and self-doubt, accomplish goals, and live a more fulfilling life. As simple as it sounds, the five second rule works by counting backwards from five to one and then simply doing the thing you want to do. In summary, the book helps people take the right course of action, instead of procrastinating or getting distracted by worry.

When I first started working on my BSR, I was practicing a similar technique, but instead of counting backwards, I counted upwards, from one to three. After reading Mel's book, I realized two things:

1. As simple and as childish as this trick might sound, not only is it effective, but it's actually based on solid behavioral science.

2. Counting backwards (three, two one) instead of counting forward (one, two, three) works even better!

The reason counting backwards works better is because counting forwards gives you room for excuses and negotiation, since once you reach three or five, you can keep counting!

"One, two, three…oh well, I'm not ready yet, I'll get up on ten. Four, five, six, seven, eight, nine, ten…" And then you're snoring!

Counting backwards is more definitive, since there's nowhere else to go after you reach one. Think about it. If you had to make a dangerous jump, what would motivate you more? Counting upwards, or counting downwards? If you were on one of those abandoned island TV shows and had to eat something really gross, how would you count—upwards, or downwards? You'll see that deep down you already know what works best.

Counting backwards before doing something is a form of metacognition, meaning it is a way of tricking your brain into doing something. It's something we've done instinctively since we were kids, like when we jumped from a tall springboard into a swimming pool!

Also, by counting backwards the moment you wake up, you give yourself your first easy task to accomplish.

This way you take advantage of the automaticity factor, and you begin building momentum for your BSR. You're also keeping yourself occupied while the primal lazy part of your brain is trying to lure you back into bed again or make you tap on the snooze button.

Although I also tried Mel's model, counting backward from five, I find that this is too long in the morning. It's long enough to give your lizard brain enough time to start making excuses. In my experience, counting backwards from three is a lot more effective when it comes to acting on something the moment you wake up. The key to this tip is taking off immediately once you reach one. The moment the countdown ends, your feet should be planted on the floor, and you should start moving away from your bed as if there's a bomb beneath it about to detonate!

You can count slowly if you want, or you can count quickly. Personally, I like a slow, steady count that starts during the exhalation part of a deep breath. You can try whatever pace works for you, but the most important thing is that you keep your mornings as identical as possible. Be as serious as the NASA guy doing the countdown during a space shuttle launch!

Ready?

Three... Two... One... Lift off!

STEP #2: QUICK MISE EN PLACE

Although I've often seen morning-routine books, articles and celebrities recommend that you start doing push-ups the moment you step out of bed, this is not a smart idea.

Your body needs to wake up, first of all, and then warm up properly if you want to get a decent workout in, so don't start banging out push-ups right away (more on this in Part 3).

Right now, all I want you to do is build momentum by getting some simple tasks out of the way—little things you'd do or like to do anyway at some point in the morning.

So, after you turn on a light or open some curtains, visit the WC, and splash some water on your face, find a few simple things to do that will keep you busy and on your feet for the next few minutes. This will help you avoid being lured back into bed by your lizard brain as your prefrontal cortex is still waking up. Do this for at least five minutes before moving to the next step.

Making the bed is one of the best tasks you can incorporate at this point. Did you know that according to a National Sleep Foundation survey, a made bed contributes to healthier sleep habits and better rest? It's also a good idea, since it'll make you think twice about trying to get back into bed again. But, if your partner is still sleeping, I also find that tidying anything else during this step has a similar effect. What works for me is washing any leftover dishes from the previous day or tidying my office.

STEP #3: HYDRATION AND/OR BREAKFAST

We all know morning hydration is important; yet, like a lot of basic things we know are good for us, we often ignore it. This is why your BSR is the perfect place to include this habit. You can make yourself a cup of coffee with a glass of water on the side. You can have a cup of your favorite tea. Or, if you're not a coffee or tea person, you can mix water with other things that will boost the taste: lemon, ginger, maybe a pinch of Himalayan salt, etc. It doesn't really matter, as long as you get some H_2O in your system and make morning hydration part of your BSR.

Deciding whether you'll be having something to eat prior to training depends on the person. Some people enjoy training fasted, while others need to eat something in order to perform. We'll be covering this in detail in Part 3. For now, keep in mind that if you do need something to eat, it has to be very light and easily digestible, since we'll be training in about twenty to thirty minutes.

You can have your morning drink and breakfast in silence and enjoy the morning peace. You can read or listen to an audiobook. You can listen to some music, some relaxing radio, or your favorite podcast. Whatever the case, remember that you want to avoid anything stressful or overstimulating. Don't worry—the world will not implode if you don't check the news, and people will not unfriend you if you don't log in and respond to their comments at 7 in the morning.

As we already covered in-depth, stuff like social media, work email, and the news are not an optimal choice, so set those aside for later. This is your personal time of the day, so find a relaxing way to enjoy your morning beverage as your prefrontal cortex is completing its start-up process.

Sidenote: If you're wondering about caffeine and dehydration, since these have been linked in the past, you can check out the Q&A section where I cover this in detail.

STEP #4: SUIT UP

The final step of your BSR is putting on your workout clothes, or what I like to call suiting-up! Even if you don't feel ready to train yet, as simple as it may sound, putting on your workout clothes can make a significant difference in getting you mentally prepped for exercise. According to a survey taken by two thousand people who exercised consistently, 88 percent of them reported that the simple act of putting on their workout clothes provided the biggest surge of motivation.

Seventy-nine percent also believed that owning good exercise clothes is an important first step toward accomplishing your fitness goals. So, even if you don't feel motivated to train yet, wait until you wear your favorite set of workout clothes to see how you feel.

Hey, maybe you can even try positive brain-conditioning by treating yourself with a set of new training clothes or a t-shirt that you only wear for your morning workout routine!

STEP #5: TUNE UP (OPTIONAL)

I actually like combining this step with the previous one by having my favorite morning workout playlist already playing as I'm suiting up. But since some people prefer training in silence, I've separated these two steps and kept the latter optional. So, feel free to figure out what works best for you!

Here's my approach: I have a standard morning playlist that I put on to set the mood. Although the list gets updated over time, I only add positive and uplifting songs to it. I find that starting every day with the same playlist creates a Pavlovian response which instantly gets me into a workout mood. If you'd like to check out my list and all the supplementary materials such as video tutorials, additional morning workout routines, and other helpful information I'll be mentioning across the book, you can find it all at www.the7AMworkoutedge.com and at the end of the book.

So, right after doing some MEP, I put on my playlist and start suiting up. I'll shamelessly admit here that I often dance a bit while putting on my boxers and shirt. Hey, don't judge me; I've got moves! Well, not really—but who cares?

Setting Up Your Own BSR

For some people, as little as fifteen minutes might be enough to get out of sleep inertia, while others need up to thirty minutes. This is something you'll figure out by yourself. I'm somewhere in the middle, since I've found that my sweet spot is twenty-five minutes.

Here's a detailed overview of how my twenty-five-minute BSR looks as I'm writing this part of the book:

1. 3-2-1 lift off!

2. Wash face with cold water.

3. Wash dishes.

4. Make coffee.

5. Enjoy coffee and favorite podcast.

6. Brush teeth.

7. Tune up & suit-up.

Each morning, after the alarm clock goes off, I take a deep breath and slowly and steadily count backwards from three. Once I reach one, I plant my feet on the floor and get moving. I know that if I manage to get up without wasting a single minute snoozing or engaging in any other point-less activity in bed, the hardest part is over! This gives me momentum, but I also try to keep in mind that my lizard brain can still take charge the moment I get side-tracked from my BSR, so I move quickly to the bathroom and splash some cold water on my face.

Next, I move to the kitchen, set the water boiler on to make some coffee, and start washing last night's leftover dishes while my coffee is getting ready. I pour myself a nice cup of fresh java, and I sit on a kitchen barstool. I avoid the couch, since I know that lying back on some comfortable cushions is still dangerous. I usually enjoy my coffee while listening to my favorite goofy podcast.

This is probably one of my favorite pockets of personal time of the day. I usually put a ten-minute timer on my phone to make sure I don't get carried away. Next, I brush my teeth, put on my morning music playlist, suit up, and begin warming up.

I move smoothly through each step, orchestrating my morning routine and preparing for my workout while keep-ing all the Mise en Place principles in my mind. Knowing that everything is planned as efficiently as possible, but also has some wiggle-room in case something unexpected gets in my way, eliminates stress and gives me clarity and confidence to begin my day.

Refining Your BSR through Time

After you figure out your own custom BSR, it is essential that you perform it in the exact same order each morning. The more you do so, the more effortless and the more ingrained it will become in your daily routine. Eventually, it will feel as simple as flipping a switch that sets you up for a great day. Don't take my word for this. Instead, my challenge for you today is to create your own BSR, stick to it for the next one and a half months, and see what happens!

All you need to do is take a piece of paper and make a list based on the guidelines above. If you have awful handwriting skills like me, printing it out is also a good idea. Although having a digital list on your smartphone as a backup is okay, I highly recommend that you use something more tangible such as paper. After all, we'll be also working on minimizing smartphone use during that first hour of the day. So, write down or print your list on paper, and keep it next to your bed, in the bathroom, or in the kitchen for daily review.

Lastly, feel free to make minor adjustments to your list during the first week; but after that, try to stick to a fixed version of it for the remaining sixty days. Each step should be clear and not more than a line of text or fifty characters. You can always make adjustments to it later on, that's okay. Over time, and as life brings about changes, tweaking and refining your BSR every now and then will become part of the process. But, always keep our five main steps as the backbone that forms your list.

Remember, the smoother the passage you create for your morning routine, the easier it will be to turn it into an effortless habit. To paraphrase Greg McKeown and his excellent book *Essentialism*, you want to "Eliminate the non-essential and make the essential frictionless."

PART 3

MORNING EXERCISE

INTRODUCTION

After my accident, I had to spend the next six years either recovering from one surgery or preparing for the next one. As I grew mentally drained and borderline depressed, my eating habits became worse and worse. I didn't eat a lot, but when I did, I cared more about amusing my taste buds and less about getting some real nutrients into my system. Alcohol and junk food would always be the more appealing choices. Even though I was in great shape before, as you can imagine, that wasn't the case anymore after close to six years of inactivity and a bad diet. So, I ended up with what we call in the fitness world a "skinny-fat physique."

When I decided to get back in shape, my resources were limited. I didn't have any personal equipment, and going to the gym wasn't an option for me for a lot of reasons. For starters, it wasn't practical, since the closest establishment was about two kilometers away, I didn't have a means of transportation, and walking big distances wasn't yet something I could do. Next, there was the social aspect of it. I had spent the last years having very few social interactions. Let's say that other than some very close friends, I avoided big crowds. I was left with social anxiety during my first years of getting back to normal life. I always was more of an introvert, but this made things a lot worse. Finally, the gym also was an extra expense that I'd rather not add until I could start earning a living again.

So, I decided to train at home, just doing basic bodyweight stuff. I did push-ups, leg raises, and all kinds of basic bodyweight exercises. As I grew stronger, I used a door frame that had a wide ledge I could hang from to do pull-ups. Combined with a healthy diet, I began to see some pretty decent results. So, I decided to put my degree in sports science to use and start working on designing my own plans, seeing how I could take things to the next level with plain old traditional calisthenics!

Similarly, you'll learn how to train in the most optimal and efficient way, through a short yet also dense and dynamic workout that will energize your body and boost your cognitive performance and mood during the rest of the day—a workout that will give you all the essential mental and physical benefits exercise can offer, in less than thirty-five minutes!

CHAPTER 8

CALISTHENICS

"If we could give every individual the right amount of nour-ishment and exercise, not too little and not too much, we would have found the safest way to health."

—HIPPOCRATES

BACK IN 2012, CALISTHENICS WEREN'T YET AS POPULAR AS THEY ARE nowadays. You mostly had people on YouTube practicing a more skill-oriented form of calisthenics that included a lot of impressive moves such as levers, muscle-ups, human flags, etc. But unless you had a ten-year background in gymnastics, these more flashy and acrobatic types of exercises seemed to be out of reach for the average person. Especially for someone who was sedentary for years and had just gone through major surgery.

There was probably only one book back then that offered a more down-to-earth approach for out-of-shape rookies like me, and so I felt that there needed to be more basic and well-designed beginner calisthenics content made available. It would be content for everyday people who simply wanted to set up a bodyweight-training routine and not train as if they're preparing for an urban calisthenics contest. That's when I realized what I wanted to do in life: I wanted to be a bodyweight coach!

I wanted to be a coach that helped the average Joe like me change his or her life through exercise and calisthenics! So, I built my first website, a YouTube channel; I also started my first company and brand: Bodyweight Muscle. And I started writing books that, to my amazement, climbed to the top of best-selling fitness-related categories on Amazon.com.

I did research, I experimented, and I kept creating new routines and figuring out ways to make the best use of the only barbell I ever used from that point: my own body.

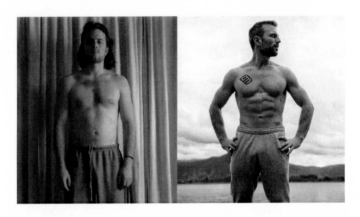

On the left of the photo above you can see a picture I took the first day before starting my journey into calisthenics. On the right, you can see me nowadays, seven years later, training mainly with my own body. No barbells, no special machines, no gym memberships.

Just to be clear, I'm not trying to promote calisthenics as *the* way. To quote *The Mandalorian* (a *Star Wars*-related TV series), although "this is the way" for me, I am not by any means a calisthenics zealot. The main purpose of this book is to show you how to take any form of exercise that is your preference and turn it into a consistent habit that helps you create your own custom morning workout edge.

So, on one hand I will indeed spend some time tooting my own "calisthenics horn," since this is the area I specialize in, and I believe a lot of people on this path can benefit from it. On the other hand, though, I'll also give you general guidelines on how to design workouts that are short and effective, no matter what kind of training you prefer.

Why Calisthenics?

The word *calisthenics* comes from the ancient Greek words kalos (κάλλος) and sthenos (σθένος). Kalos means beauty, which refers to the pleasure given by the sight of a very aesthetic human body. Sthenos is a form of mental strength that combines courage, bravery, and determination.

Since calisthenics can refer to different training systems, here's my personal view and how I define the word. For starters, I want to be clear that I'm not referring to the urban type of calisthenics (UC) that include more advanced and gymnastics-oriented skills such as muscle-ups, bars spins, levers, etc. These exercises involve highly explosive repetitive movements that multiply the tension your joints and connective tissues must absorb, which increases chances for acute and long-term overuse-related injuries—which are very common.

Although urban calisthenics are impressive, I consider them more of a sport than a fitness system for the average person like me and you. I believe that, like most sports, they're not for everyone. When it comes to the way I approach calisthenics and the training system I've spent the last ten years developing, my bodyweight training philosophy could be summarized as follows.

The Bodyweight-Muscle Definition of Calisthenics: *Calisthenics should teach you how to use your own body to develop relative strength,* *speed, and mobility in a way that is as respectful as possible to your joints and connective tissues. It's about creating a simple and practical long-term approach for staying fit, lean, and healthy that can also be sustainable and adaptable as you grow older.*

Learning to train by using your body as your main barbell is liberating. It gives you a tremendous feeling of independence. Once again, I'm not against lifting weights. Hey, if you prefer getting your morning workout edge at the gym, that's great. But I highly recommend that you learn to train with your own body, as well. That way, you'll always have a reliable option to train anywhere and anytime, no matter what the circumstances are.

No matter what's happening in the world, whether it's epidemics, pandemics, zombie apocalypses, or whatever might come our way, we can always get a workout in! By the way, I remember saying things like these prior to 2020, before the Covid-19 pandemic. I probably sounded like a calisthenics nut to some—but life is always full of surprises!

When you train with bodyweight, all you need is a room or the outdoors. You can train from the comfort of your own home; your gym can be less than a ten-second

---

*Relative strength refers to the amount of strength one has compared to his/her body weight.

commute to the living room, the garden, your garage, or the basement. There's no need to adjust to someone else's opening hours or to get stuck in traffic, waste time looking for a parking spot, or wait for your favorite machine to be available. There's no need for organizing big gym-bags and dealing with smelly, damp clothes when you unpack later on.

With morning calisthenics, it's just you, your favorite music, and the sunrise. Once you're done, you can hit the shower, prepare yourself a nice healthy breakfast, and bam— you're ready to kick off the day. Still, although this is what works for me and the people I coach, it's not something I'm trying to force on you. When it comes to selecting the type of training you'll be doing each morning, what is most important is that you pick something *you* enjoy and find practical, whether that's calisthenics, running, swimming, yoga, lifting weights, or just going for a power-walk and knocking out some push-ups in between!

Setting up Your Home Calisthenics Gym

As we've covered so far, even if you're a weight-training person, and even if you enjoy training at the gym, having a minimal calisthenics home gym setup is always a good idea. Especially at the beginning, when you're first establishing a morning workout routine, being able to train from the comfort of your own home makes things a lot easier.

To get started with setting up your home gym, let's first talk about location. You want to avoid setting up your gym next to anybody else's bedroom who will be still sleeping while you train. As quiet as you try to be in the morning, it's easy to make noise when the rest of your surroundings are peaceful. If there isn't a room in your home that is a bit secluded from other peoples' bedrooms, the garage, a backyard, or a next-door park can also be great alternatives. But you'll still need to have a setup that is convenient and usable, regardless of weather conditions like cold or rain. Personally, I like training outdoors most of the year, but I also have a home gym for extreme weather conditions such as extremely low temperatures and rain.

Equipment

Okay, time to talk about equipment. What does one need for a minimal bodyweight gym? Luckily, not a lot! In my opinion, you don't really need a lot more than a decent yoga mat and a few square feet of space to get started. Keep in mind that I'll include supplemental material at the end of the book, such as links to calisthenics morning workout routines, including a zero-equipment routine for you to get started with. I do recommend getting some extra stuff later on, though, if you feel you want to step it up a bit. For example, having something to hang from, such as a pull-up bar, is the first thing I recommend investing in. After that, it depends on your space and budget. Here are your top four options and combinations, whether you want to invest in some extra equipment right at the beginning or later on.

OPTION #1: PULL-UP BAR $–$$

If you can only invest in a single piece of equipment, start here. A simple doorway pull-up bar is the cheapest and least invasive solution. You can find a quality doorway pull-up bar nowadays for less than sixty dollars. This was my first piece of calisthenics equipment. I definitely got my money's worth, since I used it repetitively during my first four years without anything happening to it. The doorframe I hung it on did start to have some degeneration through the years, though, which is something you might want to take into consideration.

A wall-mounted pull-up bar, on the other hand, is sturdier and safer—but also a more expensive and invasive option. In summary, if it fits your budget and you have a sturdy wall to drill on, I highly recommend one of the wall-mounted options. Otherwise, go for the doorway pull-up bar.

OPTION #2: GYMNASTIC RINGS $

This is my favorite option, but it is also a more invasive option, since you'll probably have to drill eye bolts into your ceiling. But, it will cost you almost the same as a doorframe pull-up bar while offering you a much broader exercise repertoire. The reason I love gymnastic rings is because they are a pull-up bar, a dip station, and a suspension trainer all in one! Gymnastic rings are always my faithful workout companion—I never train without them! Especially if you enjoy training outdoors, they are a no-brainer. When the weather is good, and you have extra time, you can always easily remove them from your home setup, throw them in your backpack, and use them to train at your favorite outdoor spot.

There are a few ways to set up your rings indoors, and the first thing to do is ensure that your anchor point(s) can withstand your weight—safety comes first! Most times, installing heavy-duty eye bolts on the ceiling is the safest and sturdiest solution. Some less invasive options you can consider for setting up your gymnastic rings are sturdy objects you can hang them around such as rafters, beams, or an exposed joist on an unfinished ceiling you might have in your garage or attic.

OPTION #3: PULL-UP BAR + GYMNASTIC RINGS COMBO $$

If you want to be able to perform a wider variety of calisthenics exercises without having to drill anything indoors, this combo is probably the best way to go for intermediate and advanced calisthenics trainees. It is a more expensive option, but it allows you to perform all the essential bodyweight exercises such as pull-ups, inverted rows, and gymnastic ring dips. Still, this might not be an ideal combination for beginners, since exercises such as dips are not that easy to learn on gymnastic rings—although I will once again include progressions in extra resources at the end of the book. This is why I recommend the next option for beginners and those willing to invest a bit more on equipment.

OPTION #4: PULL-UP BAR AND DIP STATION $$$

An even sturdier and a more preferable solution for beginner calisthenics trainees is combining a pull-up bar and a dip station. A dip station is a great tool to do multiple exercises such as dips and inverted rows. I prefer dip stations that connect into a single, solid piece, since dip stations that consist of independent parallettes are usually too unstable. A proper dip station is not cheap, but it's a great piece of equipment to have, especially if you're a beginner calisthenics trainee and you want to master classic bodyweight exercises.

WHAT ABOUT PULL-UP TOWERS?

I've owned and tried various pull-up towers in the past. Personally, I find them too impractical, mainly due to their size—especially if you live in an apartment. They end up taking up space, they are difficult to move, and the ones that are light are usually too unstable. Lastly, they are also too expensive. If you have the budget, I recommend spending it on one of the options above.

PARALYSIS BY ANALYSIS

Don't spend too much time obsessing about equipment. Rather, focus on the minimum things you need to get started. Tony Robbins says that success is not about resources, but about resourcefulness! Apply this mindset to your training, and you'll see that there are no limits to what you can accomplish through calisthenics! When you see your body as the main barbell that you have mastered using in order to get in great shape, you can always find a way to train no matter where you are! A lack of equipment is simply an opportunity to be a bit more creative, whether that's at your home gym, a park, or in a hotel room during a business trip. So, don't end up overwhelmed trying to decide which is the perfect piece or combination of equipment for you. Give it no more than fifteen minutes of thought, pick one of the options above, and get started!

CHAPTER 9

HIGH-FREQUENCY TRAINING BENEFITS

"If it's important, do it every day. If it's not important, don't do it at all…"
—DAN GABLE

MOST PEOPLE AIM TO HAVE TWO OR THREE LONG AND ENERGY-DEPLETING workouts per week. The benefit of high-frequency training is that your training volume can be spread optimally across the week through daily short and rejuvenating workouts that don't have to last more than thirty-five minutes!

By training every day, I mean working out a minimum of five days per week. I also recommend that all of your workouts are done on work days! In summary, for most people this means training from Monday to Friday or Saturday. Never make a busy workday an excuse to not work out because that's how most people begin to fall off the wagon!

When you train every day, the truth is that you don't need more than thirty minutes on average of quality work to get and stay in good shape! I get it if you might feel skeptical about this and if it might sound too good to be true, since a lot of us in the past have spent hours in the gym with very little to show for it.

Yet, if you compared a focused, high-quality workout with a workout where so much time is spent socializing, waiting in turn for our favorite workout machine to be free, procrastinating on our phone, doing exercises that do very little for us, looking at the attractive trainee next to us, and, in general, all the time spent *not* focused on the training itself, then it will make sense!

Our mind is extremely talented at wasting time, especially during challenging tasks such as working out. This is why, during Part 1 of the book, we focused on setting up a morning routine that doesn't leave a lot of room for distractions and procrastination!

Once you get in the zone and you make every second of your sessions count, not only will your workouts be more efficient, but you'll also enjoy them more. Before you know it, the workout will be over, and you'll be looking forward to the next day's session. And that, my friend, is one of the biggest secrets to creating a consistent, enjoyable routine: always finish your session fresh and feeling you'd like to do a bit more! This way you'll stay "hungry" for the next session, and training will never feel like a chore.

Last, but not least, you'll always finish your training left with an abundance of energy, which, combined with all the mood-boosting chemicals in your body, will carry over to the rest of your day!

If It's Important, Do It Every Day

When you start trying to figure out which are the ideal days to train based on your work schedules, your workload, when you'll be feeling the least tired, etc., then you never end up with a consistent workout routine! This requires too much effort and planning—which, as we've already established so many times in the book, gives your mind room for negotiation! The 7 A.M. Workout Edge is not something you do when you have enough time or energy; it's something you start each day with *because* it generates more energy and time! Your morning routine should be part of your lifestyle, no matter what's going on during the rest of your day. It becomes something you do on a daily basis and something that is as unquestionable as brushing your teeth or taking a shower (I hope). This way, you leave no room for excuses!

Just as professional athletes have their pre-game rituals, you can turn your morning workout edge into your pre-day ritual! It can be something you start each morning with, knowing how much better you'll perform during the rest of the day because of it. Even on days when you struggle a bit to get started, knowing that things will always be better once you get your morning workout in is the secret of the 7 A.M. Workout Edge! It is why people who train in the morning consider exercise part of their lifestyle and not just a simple habit.

Exercise is a benefit you experience instantly, whereas training for a long-term goal such as fat loss and building your ideal physique are both goals that are too far away in the future. This often makes them too vague to keep you motivated in the moment and on a daily basis. Sure, long-term goals are important, but I consider these more like the long-term positive side-effects of the morning workout edge. Knowing that once you complete your workout you'll be setting yourself up for a great day is always a much stronger motive to have during your workout!

Simply said, if it's important, you'll do it every day.

Performance and Body Composition

Now that we've covered the important parts of the 7 A.M. Workout Edge, we can also talk about performance and aesthetics. After all, who doesn't want to be in great shape and look good in front of a mirror?

High-frequency training has been one of the key aspects of my workout approach and getting in great shape. For starters, training every day allows me to focus on quality over quantity. Think about it like this: how many sets until failure can you get per exercise if you warm-up well in a single workout? For example, if you went all-in and tried to break your own pull-up record? I would say no more than one set. Some could argue two sets, but that would require a huge resting period, making your workout too long.

Sure, you can train a specific exercise or muscle group once or twice a week as a lot of people do, trying to cram all your weekly training volume into those two sessions. But, spreading that volume over five to six short workouts (especially if you want to keep your workouts short) allows you to capitalize on quality over quantity and maximize your results when it comes to building muscle and strength. After having tried all kinds of different training frequencies over the years, my greatest results in terms of body composition and performance have come from high-frequency training.

No, I'm not a high frequency training zealot, and I don't believe that high-frequency is the only way to get in good shape. But, in my experience—especially when it comes to a sustainable morning routine, and people who have a challenging weekly schedule due to work and other responsibilities—high frequency training seems to offer the best results while also being the most practical solution.

Staying Fit after Thirty, Forty, Fifty, and Sixty

Satellite cells are those that are responsible for muscle memory and muscle-mass maintenance, but they can also speed up muscle growth. These cells start to decrease as we age past our thirties, and high frequency training is one of the best ways to keep them alive! As shown in a scientific paper titled "Satellite Cells in Aging: Use It or Lose It," researchers concluded that people need to activate their muscles on a regular basis once they reach age thirty or face the possibility of losing the ability to regenerate muscle mass as they age, making regular exercise all the more important for people as they grow older.

Those of us closer to forty or fifty than thirty know that a week of letting go is enough to start feeling out of shape. The body feels heavier, more clunky, and cumbersome. Other than being demotivating, I also believe that this is a sign from our body, telling us that we can't afford to spread our workouts too far apart from each other if we want to maintain our fitness momentum. One of the biggest and most important realizations I've made in the last decade is that the best way to preserve muscle mass, stay in shape, promote longevity, and overall feel great as you get older is figuring out how to get the smallest and most efficient dose of exercise on a daily basis.

How to Structure Your Workout Week

As I've already said, what is most important is that you find a weekly workout structure that makes you happy, whether that means jogging every day, having a yoga routine, or jumping on a trampoline! Still, since a lot of you might be looking for suggestions and ideas, here's a blueprint of my weekly routine.

On Mondays, Wednesdays, and Fridays I always make sure I do my calisthenics (strength-training) workout. On Tuesdays and Thursdays, I'll do hill sprints. And, since I like to have no structure on Saturdays, I'll just do whatever feels right during that day. Oftentimes, this will be a thirty-minute jog; other times, it might be a calisthenics routine; and sometimes, it can be another planned group activity such as hiking! As long as I'm active during my Saturday, I'm happy with whatever I end up doing.

- **Monday:** calisthenics

- **Tuesday:** hill sprints

- **Wednesday:** calisthenics

- **Thursday:** hill sprints

- **Friday:** calisthenics

- **Saturday:** jogging, calisthenics, hiking, or anything that keeps me active

CHAPTER 10

THE WARM-UP IS THE HARDEST PART

"To be prepared is half the victory."
—MIGUEL DE CERVANTES

MERELY BY WATCHING SOMEONE WARM UP, I CAN TELL IF HE OR SHE HAS A consistent workout plan. A proper warm-up is the cornerstone of any successful long-term workout routine. A proper warm-up helps you prevent injury and increases performance, which can also help you get better results from your training. Even though most of us are aware of all this, the warm-up still remains one of the most boring parts of working out and usually one that we'd rather skip—especially when we're young and our bodies feel indestructible.

But, even though we might feel that we can beat our body down with seemingly no repercussions at the time, we eventually start to pay for all that abuse from the past. Trust me, things that feel like mild discomfort and seem innocent when you're twenty-two will eventually come back to bite you in the butt!

There comes a point though, usually somewhere after your early thirties (if not earlier), where you begin to see the big picture. You realize that the body can only take so much beating up until things start to break down slowly. Being meticulous with your warm-up is a one-way road if you want to keep exercise as part of your life as you grow older.

Warm-Up and the Workout Is Over

Besides the physical benefits of warming up properly, there is another reason why you want to master your warm-up routine no matter how old you are. Having a standard warm-up routine is an essential workout when it comes to jump-starting your motivation to exercise—especially during days when willpower is on the low end of the spectrum!

I mentioned this a bit during Part 1 of the book, but it's also worth mentioning again—the most challenging thing during days you're not in the mood to exercise is not the actual workout—it's everything else that precedes it! It's all those little actions of preparation prior to training that cause most of the mental friction. And if waking up is the first, stickiest point of your morning routine, the second one tends to be the warm-up!

Most people think that the hardest part of working out is the main part of the workout that requires the most physical effort. In reality, the hardest and stickiest part is the warm-up! If this doesn't make any sense to you, try to be mindful of it the next time you're struggling to begin your workout. You'll realize that if you manage to move past the warm-up, you'll always have enough momentum to keep going. Before you know it, you're blasting reps, listening to your favorite tune, and all the initial struggle has faded away. I've never seen anyone quit a workout due to a lack of motivation once they're past their warm-up!

If you can remember one thing from this second part of the book, it should be this: if you manage to get yourself to warm up, you can consider the workout done!

In one of my favorite books on habits, *Tiny Habits*, Brian Fogg calls these actions "starter steps." A starter step is the first step in a longer sequence of behaviors. For example, opening your sketchbook is a starter step in drawing a picture. Setting an apple on the kitchen counter is a starter step for eating more fruit. Warming up, just like putting on your exercise clothes, are both starter steps for working out.

Starter steps remove mental friction and the brain's tendency to make excuses when it feels intimidated by a complex task. It's like tricking yourself. The next time you don't feel like working out, give this a try. Simply tell yourself "I'll just warm-up and see how I feel." Don't start by trying to commit to the whole workout. When motivation is low, this will only make you feel overwhelmed! Simply commit to getting in your warm-up. Surprisingly, you'll see that not only will you go all the way, but a lot of times, you'll even have one of your best sessions!

THE TWO KEYS FOR TURNING YOUR WARM-UP INTO A STARTER STEP

The two keys to making your warm-up routine an effective starter step are the following:

1. Find a good one first (not too long, not too short).

2. Marry this routine for the next one and a half months.

Your morning warm-up shouldn't be so long that it ends up being overwhelming during days that motivation is low, but also not so short that it's ineffective. You should learn it by heart, to the extent that you can perform it while thinking about other random things. It should become as automatic as the rest of your BSR's habits.

Warming Up in the Morning versus Warming Up in the Afternoon

One of the biggest mistakes people make when it comes to morning exercise is training the same way they would train in the afternoon. This often leads to workouts that feel stiff, clunky, and, in the end, disappointingly unproductive!

Your muscles, tendons, and ligaments need to be treated differently in the morning after being inactive for so many hours. Compared to an afternoon workout, your body needs at least thirty percent more warming up during the first hours after you're awake. Still, spending thirty minutes just to warm-up in the morning is not a luxury most adults with busy schedules have.

Plus, it's something that can be intimidating for those new to morning exercise, but also boring for anyone in the long run. In summary, most of us usually don't want to spend half of our morning warming up. Ideally, we want to get started as quickly as possible and have a workout that is short, enjoyable, and effective.

Right?

This is why not only will I share with you how to master your morning warm-up, but also how to adapt your workouts in a way that intensity is built in gradually.

Is Static Stretching Good for Warming Up in the Morning?

Static stretching is an important part of the warm-up that I'll be sharing with you in the next chapter. Since this has become quite a controversial topic in the last decade, I wanted to share my thoughts on it.

Back when I was growing up, everyone had to stretch before practice and games to improve performance and prevent injury. It was considered common knowledge. Then, about twenty-something years ago, studies began to suggest that stretching could actually be bad for performance and even increase injury risk, creating widespread confusion that persists today. I admit it: being someone who always found stretching extremely boring, I jumped on that train simply because it suited me.

After having studied this topic deeper and also after having found the value behind my morning stretches, I can't imagine starting my morning warm-up any other day. Although my younger self would cringe if he heard me say this, I admit that I've learned to love morning static stretches!

As usually happens in the exercise science world, the problem is that people who were behind those studies that "framed" static stretching as the bad guy examined stretching in a vacuum. So, after using excessive static-stretching routines as the only means of warming up, it makes sense that the researchers got the results they got (or were looking for).

Sure, if excessive static stretching is the only thing you do to warm up, then yes, you might be even doing more bad than good for both injury prevention and performance.

But, if you carefully review research on this topic you'll realize that static stretching can actually be an important part of a complete warm-up if it's properly sequenced and combined with more dynamic exercises. Particularly when it comes to morning workouts, I consider light static-stretching essential!

If you don't want to take my word for it, you can check out Dr. David G. Behm (University Research Professor at the School of Human Kinetics and Recreation, Memorial University of Newfoundland, Canada) and his colleague's work. What they found after a review of hundreds of studies was that static stretching combined with an initial warm-up and some dynamic stretching—which involves actively moving muscles through their range of motion, as in walking lunges or torso twists—followed by sport-specific activities, such as swinging a baseball bat, can improve performance and reduce injury risk. Of the reliable studies in the review that looked specifically at injuries, there was "a 54 percent risk reduction in acute muscle injuries associated with stretching," the researchers wrote in 2016 in the *Journal of Applied Physiology, Nutrition, and Metabolism*.

Why Light Static Stretching in the Morning Is Good for You

When it comes to static stretching, think of your neuro-muscular system (NMS) as a protective mechanism. When you make a sudden move that involves a range of motion (ROM) that your body is not used to (especially early in the morning) this protective mechanism overreacts by keeping your muscles and, by proximity, their surrounding connective tissues tight. It also sometimes overreacts by reflexively keeping areas tight due to old injuries or fear of new movement patterns. Yes, as counterintuitive as it sounds, it's your NMS that prevents you from being flexible, not your muscles being "short," which is what a lot of people think! Light static stretching is the first step in helping your body loosen up and increase your range of motion.

In summary, when it comes to morning static stretching, you want to keep it short (keep it below a minute) and always stretch to the point of mild discomfort—you don't have to overdo it (the more you relax your whole body while in that sweet spot of mild discomfort, the deeper your stretch will become)!

CHAPTER 11

THE PERFECT MORNING WARM-UP ROUTINE

"The warm-up is the workout."
—DAN JOHN

FROM A TECHNICAL PERSPECTIVE, THE GOALS OF THE WARM-UP THAT I'll be sharing with you are to increase mobility, range of motion, and overall performance while minimizing the chances of any potential injury that might occur while working out.

For starters, we use static stretches that loosen up the neuromuscular system, which tends to keep the body stiff, especially early in the morning. And next, we use more dynamic movements that mobilize all the main segments of the spine (cervical, thoracic, and lumbar), lubricate the joints with synovial fluid (think of this as your joint's natural grease), and increase blood flow to your limbs and the rest of the body's periphery.

Although this is what any decent warm-up should do for you before engaging in intense physical exercise, I see this morning warm-up routine as something that offers much more than just that.

It's a routine that I've been refining for years, looking for the "best bang for your buck" exercises, and combining them in the most efficient way possible, to create the shortest and most dense routine one can do in the morning—not only to prepare for a dynamic workout ahead, but to also to gain a more holistic effect of physical wellness.

This routine helps you to:

1. Decompress from the toll that bad posture and excessive sitting might have put on your body the previous day.

2. Shake off that stiff and clunky morning sensation your body wakes up with.

3. Start moving as gracefully and as effortlessly as possible during the rest of the day.

In summary, if I could recommend one morning routine for overall physical wellness, this would be it! Once you go through it, you should move and feel almost as supple and as confident as Muhammad Ali before a boxing match in his prime! You should be ready to face the rest of the day with a feeling of "I can float like a butterfly and sting like a bee!"

Before I start describing the routine, keep two things in mind.

For starters, although I've done my best to explain all the exercises below, I've also created a detailed video demonstration for you, which you'll find a link to at the end of the book (or by visiting www.the7AMworkoutedge.com

now). I recommend going through the guidelines below once, and then having your phone play next to you as you go through the routine.

Lastly, also take into consideration that until you get a good handle on it, the routine might initially take you some extra time to complete. Therefore, I say put aside twenty minutes for each session, simply to be able to practice it stress-free. Don't worry if this feels too long at first. It's only a matter of time until you master the routine and learn to execute it in almost half that time. Once you learn everything by heart and you start transitioning faster and smoother from one exercise to the other, you'll eventually be getting through it in no more than eleven minutes!

My Eleven-Minute Morning Warm-Up Routine

We begin our exercises on the floor, so ideally, make sure you have a nice, soft yoga mat. Starting from the top of our body (the cervical spine), we'll move gradually downwards, covering all the segments of the spine and all the main joints and muscle groups. Finally, we'll finish off with a few more exercises from a standing position.

PART 1. CERVICAL SPINE

Begin from a prone position, lying down on a soft surface. The cervical part of your spine can be quite sensitive, so always start gently and move your head smoothly.

A. NECK-EXTENSOR STRETCH (FIFTEEN SECONDS)

Lift your chest off the ground, and with your nose pointing downwards, cross your fingers behind your head and push lightly against it while keeping your elbows resting on the floor. This will stretch the typically tonic muscles of the back of the neck and lighten the load which forward-head posture puts on your cervical spine most of the day.

B. NECK ROTATION (FOUR REPS)

Gently turn your head left and right (that's one rep). Start slowly and gradually increase your range of motion little by little as you loosen up and get used to the exercise.

C. NECK FLEXION AND EXTENSION (FOUR REPS)

Bring your head backward as if you're trying to look at the sky (or ceiling) and then downwards as if you're trying to look at your sternum—that's one rep. Keep your tongue on the roof of your mouth on the way up, since this will help your neck flexors to stretch more efficiently.

PART 2. SHOULDERS

We continue from the same prone position. Make sure that you avoid hyperextension of the neck at this point. Always maintain a neutral position in the cervical segment by keeping the nose pointing downwards.

A. SHOULDER ROLLS (EIGHT REPS)

Make big and smooth backward circles with your shoulders, rolling them back and away from your body and bringing them forward again.

B. PRONE ANGELS (EIGHT TO TWELVE REPS)

Lift your torso slightly so that your chest and head are not touching the floor. Brace your glutes to keep the lower back light. Brace your quadriceps, extend your knees while keeping them off the ground, and point your toes backwards.

Now that you've assumed the right starting position, bring your arms to the front with your palms facing the floor and your elbows bent. Once your index fingers touch, move your arms backwards while rotating your palms upwards (facing the ceiling) and extending them next to your thighs—that's one rep!

PART 3. SPINE AND LOWER BODY

To transition to the next exercise, get in a quadruped position (lean on your knees and palms, as if you're a four-legged animal).

A. CAT-COW POSE (EIGHT REPS)

From this table-like pose, inhale while curving your lower back and bringing your head up, sinking your belly and tilting your pelvis anteriorly like a "cow." Next, exhale deeply and bring your abdomen in, arching your spine and bringing your head and pelvis down—getting into the typical stretch you see cats do. That's one repetition!

B. FIGURE FOUR STRETCH (TWENTY TO THIRTY SECONDS)

Our next exercise is a great stretch for the deep gluteal muscles (such as the piriformis) which tend to put pressure on your sciatic and often become problematic for lower back issues. This one can be complex when you're trying it for the first time, so let's break it down into four steps.

1. Start by lying on your back with your left knee bent and its foot flat on the floor.

2. Bring your right leg's ankle on top of your left knee (kind of like forming a figure four).

3. Reach with your right arm through your bent knee, and your left arm around your left thigh, crossing your fingers behind it.

4. Pull your left thigh backwards and towards your chest.

You should feel the stretch in the deeper gluteal layers of your right buttock. Keep the rest of the body relaxed and next repeat for the opposite side. If the stretch becomes easy, you can cross your fingers on top of your shin (instead of your thigh) for a more intense stretch.

C. LYING HIP AND GLUTE STRETCH (TWENTY TO THIRTY SECONDS)

From a supine position again, keep your shoulder blades square on the floor, and use your left hand to guide your right knee across your body and towards the floor on your left side. Maintain this position for twenty to thirty seconds and repeat for the other side.

Don't force your knee to touch the floor if your flexibility does not allow it.

D. LUMBAR ROCKS (EIGHT REPS)

This is my favorite spine and lower back mobility exercise. From the same position as above, bend your knees at about ninety degrees, with your feet flat on the floor and at an arm's-length distance from the rest of the body. Next, extend your arms like you're trying to form a capital letter T. Rock your knees to the right and left while keeping your upper body as stable as possible by maintaining your palms flat against the floor. If this is easy, you can cautiously progress to doing the same exercise with your feet in the air.

Go for eight reps in total.

E. GLUTE BRIDGES (TWELVE TO FOURTEEN REPS)

With your feet in the same position (still at an arm's-length distance and flat on the floor), press your heels against the floor and bring your pelvis to a height where knees, pelvis, and shoulders are all aligned. Squeeze the glutes at the top while making sure your pelvis is in posterior pelvic tilt (never hyperextending the lower back) and go down again.

F. LYING KNEE EXTENSIONS (TEN TO TWELVE REPS)
Next, straighten one leg on the floor and lift the other with your knee bent and your fingers crossed behind your thigh. From this position, extend your knee until you feel a light stretch in the hamstrings or calves, and return to the original bent position. This is one rep.

G. SEATED HAMSTRING STRETCH (TWENTY TO THIRTY SECONDS)
Sit with one leg extended and your other leg bent, with the sole of your foot resting against your mid-thigh. Reach towards your toes with your back straight (bent from the hip instead of hunching forward). Repeat for the other leg and next with both legs straight in front of you. Don't force yourself to grab your toes if you can't. It's okay to only go as far as your ankle, shin, or even your knees. What is most important is that you feel the stretch in your hamstrings, and you maintain proper posture.

H. SEATED WINDMILLS | DYNAMIC STATIC STRETCH (TEN REPS)
Next, open both legs in front of you at an angle you feel comfortable. Next, twist your upper body right and left, extending each hand's fingers towards the opposite foot's

toes. Keep your chest out, and never hunch forward. Even though this will decrease your range of motion, always bend at the hip. One rep counts as two opposite toe touches.

If you struggle to maintain an upright posture from the seated position described above (some people might even feel tightness in the lower back in this position) you can cheat the exercise by bending your knees as much as required to assume the proper upright position. The more you practice this whole routine, the more your movements will improve.

I. HIP AND QUAD STRETCH (TWENTY TO THIRTY SECONDS)

This is another one that often mixes up people in the beginning, so let's also break it down in steps.

1. Bring your left leg forward in a lunge position and lean with your right knee on the ground.

2. Place your hands next to your forward left foot and slightly lean forward, while maintaining your right knee anchored on the floor and your left knee at a ninety-degree angle. Keeping the right knee anchored this way will help you with properly stretching your hip flexors, which is what we're aiming for.

3. To make sure you are positioned right, always keep enough space between your two legs. Repeat for both sides.

PART 4. STANDING EXERCISES

Next, we'll move to a few more standing exercises.

A. DOORWAY CHEST STRETCH (TWENTY TO THIRTY SECONDS)

This one is great for the chest and front delts, muscles that are typically tight due to slouching in an office and overall bad posture.

Stand under a doorway and raise each arm to the side. Bend your elbows at a ninety-degree angle and rest your palms on the doorway (facing away from you). Slowly step forward with one foot until you feel a light stretch in your shoulders and chest. Stand upright and hold for thirty seconds.

B. STRAIGHT-ELBOW PUSH-UP (TEN REPS)

From a straight elbow plank position, with your knees extended and your quadriceps braced (this helps keep your pelvis from sinking), protract and retract your shoulder blades. I guess a more technical term for the exercise would be "straight-plank shoulder-blade protraction and retraction," but I think straight-elbow push-ups give a better picture of the exercise. It's very common for people to bend their elbows during this exercise, since not doing so feels weird at first. Be extra mindful to avoid doing that.

C. PASSIVE DEAD HANG (TWENTY TO THIRTY SECONDS)

The passive dead hang is the best exercise to get you out of your hunched office posture and realign your body. It stretches your lats, pecs, and biceps, and it decompresses your spine. Most importantly, though, it's one of the best exercises you can do for flexibility, mobility, and overall shoulder health, since it pulls the shoulders back into their natural alignment. It is also a great exercise to prepare your shoulders and increase their range of motion before working out.

Other than your grip and forearms, nothing else should be tight, so relax and let gravity do her thing. Aim for thirty seconds (start with less if you're a beginner), but the more you can hold without overexerting yourself the merrier. If this feels too hard in the beginning, you can also start with an easier progression by slightly leaning on the tips of your toes.

D. THE EGYPTIAN (TWELVE TO FOURTEEN REPS)

Again, from a straight standing position, extend your arms away from the body. Turn one palm up (external shoulder rotation), and at the same time, turn the other palm back (internal shoulder rotation). Next, reverse this position, and you've got one rep. The movement resembles the unwrapping of a candy a bit, which is why I also call these "candy-wrappers" when I train kids! Do a total of ten repetitions.

E. STRAIGHT-ELBOW PULL-UPS (TWELVE TO FOURTEEN REPS)

From a passive dead-hang, move to an active dead-hang and back. That's one rep. I like to call these straight-elbow pull-ups, since when you're performing them your body moves up and down while your elbows remain straight. To accomplish this, you want to slightly retract your shoulder blades (bring them together) and next depress (pull back and down), pointing your chest a bit upwards as your body rises. Move smoothly and slowly, especially on the way back down. If you're too weak to perform this exercise, focus first on achieving a thirty-second passive dead-hang and add straight-elbow pull-ups later in the mix.

F. BODYWEIGHT SQUATS (FIFTEEN REPS)

There are enough tutorials on squats online, so I won't elaborate on form here. Your goal is to gradually increase your ROM, going as deep as possible with perfect form. Aim for a number of reps that keeps effort at about forty percent. For most people, this will be between ten and fifteen repetitions.

Caution

Although this warm-up routine can improve your flexibility to some extent in the long run, it is not our main goal (our main goal is to prepare the body for working out right after)! If you want to focus on flexibility, the best time to work on it is *after* working out and later in the day.

Lastly, keep in mind that everyone has different abilities and limitations. At no point during this warm-up should you be forcing yourself to the point of extreme discomfort or pain. Always aim for a light stretch or an amount of effort that feels well within your reach. Remember, your body is still cold and has moved very little for almost half a day. Always begin each exercise very conservatively, and stay focused on your body's feedback. It will always let you know what feels right and what doesn't.

CHAPTER 12

STRENGTH TRAINING

"Without knowledge, skill cannot be focused. Without skill, strength cannot be brought to bear. And without strength, knowledge may not be applied."
—ALEXANDER THE GREAT

STRENGTH TRAINING IS ONE OF THE BEST WAYS TO GET YOUR MORNING workout edge and it is one of the best things you can do for your overall well-being in general. Here are just some of the benefits for people who strength train on a weekly basis.

- Lower risk of chronic disease

- Improved body composition (better muscle-to-fat ratio)

- Healthier bones

- Decreased blood pressure

- Lower LDL (bad) cholesterol

- Increased mobility and flexibility (contrary to popular belief, proper strength training can also increase joint range of motion)

- Increased self-efficacy (the belief that you're able to succeed at or perform a task)

- Positive body image

- Reduced anxiety

- Brain health and function

- Protection against age-related cognitive decline

- Increased pain management

The world of strength training is huge nowadays, ranging from traditional weight-lifting to CrossFit, traditional bodybuilding, calisthenics, kettlebell training, and all the new methods that keep popping up each day. Everything has become mainstream! This is great, since strength training is essential for your physical and mental health, and having a lot of different options can help people find what suits them best.

But that also makes it impossible for me to cover them all in a book like this one. So instead, I'll do my best to give you a basic framework you can adapt to whichever form of strength training you find ideal.

What is most important for you to remember is that our goal is getting the minimum effective dose of exercise that allows us to train on a daily basis.

Warming Up

If you're doing calisthenics, then the morning warm-up routine we covered in the previous chapter combined with the following guidelines will be sufficient for you. If you're doing something different, especially if you're into a strength-oriented activity that includes heavy weight-lifting, you'll want to advise your coach or trainer on adding some more targeted supplementary warm-up exercises.

Exercise Selection

To simplify things, we'll be dividing our exercises in movement patterns that cover the whole body. Since I'm a calisthenics guy, a lot of the examples I'll be offering will be in that context, but you can easily apply it to whatever form of strength training it is that you do.

1. Pull movements (e.g., pull-ups and inverted rows)

2. Push movements (e.g., pike or handstand push-ups, regular push-ups, and dips)

3. Lower-body knee-dominant movements (e.g., most squatting and lunging exercises)

4. Lower-body hip-dominant movements (e.g., glute bridges and good mornings)

5. Movement or resistance of movement generated by the core (e.g., planks, leg raises and hollow-body holds)

Every workout should cover the whole body, meaning you want to pick a pull, a push, one lower body exercise (hip- or knee-dominant), and one core exercise. If you decide to strength train every day, you want to also pick different exercise variations from day to day in order to recover efficiently.

For example, if on one day you do a vertical pull (e.g., pull-ups), then the next day, focus on a horizontal pull (e.g., inverted rows). If one day you focus on a knee-dominant lower body exercise (e.g., squats), the next day, focus on a hip-dominant exercise (e.g., hip thrusts). If one day you focus on a more horizontal push (e.g., push-ups), the next day, focus on a more vertical push (e.g., shoulder press or pike push-ups). If one day you focus on some kind of plank abdominal exercise, the next day, focus on a supine type of abdominal exercise (e.g., hollow-body holds).

Let's start with a calisthenics example.

CALISTHENICS: DAY 1

1. Pull-ups (vertical pull)

2. Wall-sit (knee-dominant lower body)

3. Push-ups (horizontal push)

4. Plank (Core exercise)

CALISTHENICS: DAY 2

1. Inverted rows (horizontal pull)

2. Glute bridges (hip-dominant lower body)

3. Pike push-ups (vertical push)

4. Hollow-body holds (Supine core exercise)

Here's a more traditional gym-workout example.

GYM WORKOUT: DAY 1

1. Lat pull-down (vertical pull)

2. Barbell squats (knee-dominant lower body)

3. Bench press (horizontal push)

4. Plank (core exercise)

GYM WORKOUT: DAY 2

1. Rowing machine (horizontal pull)

2. Barbell hip thrust (hip-dominant lower body)

3. Shoulder press (vertical push)

4. Dead-bugs (supine core exercise)

These are just some templates to help you get started with ideas on how to design your own plan. As I said, there are all kinds of different camps and schools of thought out there nowadays when it comes to training, and especially strength-training.

The purpose of this book is not to help you to design the best morning workout routine, since that can be a hugely controversial topic and would require a whole different book of its own. The purpose of this book is to help you make short morning workouts an effortless part of your morning routine. Still, if you feel you need more help in this area, you can check out some detailed calisthenic routines I find practical to do in the mornings at the end of the book.

How to Structure Your Workouts

Some people are curious about recovery when I talk about high frequency training. When it comes to strength training, there's a generalization that you can't train the same muscle groups on consecutive days. Yet, that is an outdated idea, since training frequency is not the only variable that affects recovery. Total volume, time under tension, and load are even more important factors to keep in mind. Because our workouts will be short and low in training volume, training the whole body on consecutive days is no problem.

Keeping all that in mind, I recommend that you structure your workout in three rounds. During each round, you want to cycle your exercises like a circuit, since linear training takes too much time. I also recommend alternating from upper body to lower body or core exercises, to allow yourself faster recovery from station to station.

Depending on your condition and training level, aim for fifteen to forty seconds of rest in between each exercise. Aim for the higher end (thirty to forty seconds) after exercises that create higher oxygen debt, such as plyometric exercises (e.g., box jumps, burpees, jumping rope, etc.). Aim for the lower end (fifteen to twenty seconds) after more static and low oxygen-debt exercises (e.g., pull-ups, push-ups, planks, wall-sits, etc.). The general idea is resting just enough to enter the next exercise feeling strong, while also keeping your heart rate going so you condition the cardiovascular system.

ROUND 1: GET YOUR ENGINE STARTED

During your first round, you want to go easy on your body and stay below fifty percent away from failure. In simple words, if you feel you can get ten push-ups, go for five. Think of this as more of a warm-up round.

I also recommend using a slow 3–1 tempo during your first round. That means to take three seconds to complete the negative (easy) phase and one second to complete the positive (hard) phase of each rep. For example, during a push-up, go down in three seconds and then go up again in one second. Or, during pull-ups, pull yourself up in one second, and go down again in three seconds.

This round should feel easy, and once again, you want to stay away from failure. You want enough muscle tension for your neuromuscular system to know that the workout has begun, but you also want to allow yourself to ease into things and avoid feeling stiff or clunky. Think of your body as an old car during a cold winter morning. Until the engine and all its parts are fully warmed up, you've got to take it easy and drive slow.

A minute of rest after this round should be sufficient.

ROUND 2: LEAVE 20 PERCENT IN THE TANK

During your second round, you want to switch things up a gear. You can use your regular rep tempo and get some more serious work in, but still, you want to stay away from failure. Perform each exercise with strict form and push yourself harder, but make sure you *leave a couple of reps in the tank*. Aim for about 70–80 percent of the max reps and intensity you'd usually go for during an afternoon workout. For example, if you'd typically do ten pull-ups during this round in the afternoon, go for seven to eight reps. Or, if you'd be bench pressing a hundred pounds for twelve reps during this set in the afternoon, go for seventy to eighty pounds.

Since our goal is to go all in during the following round, make sure you get enough rest before moving on. Two to three minutes should be enough.

ROUND 3: GET YOUR BEST REPS IN

By round three, your body should be all fired up for maximum performance. So if you feel ready, I recommend always aiming for technical failure during this round. In simple words, training to technical failure means getting as many reps as possible, as long as you maintain proper form. In other words, push yourself as hard as you can, as long as it's never at the expense of bad form.

When you're new to morning exercise and you try this approach, you might feel you're not getting a lot done during your first rounds. But, try to see the big picture! What's really happening during rounds one and two is that you're taking time to prepare your body, and because of that, you can perform a lot better during the last round. This way, you're still getting enough overall training volume, and, by going to failure during your last round, your body also gets enough overall intensity.

This approach allows you to keep your joints and connective tissues safe while also making the whole session feel smooth. In the end, it also allows you to finish your workout with a strong set, which gives you a boost of motivation, confidence, and energy that carries over to the rest of the day. Lastly, it also leaves you fresh and looking forward to your next morning workout where you can repeat the same process!

Of course, tweaking your reps and sets this way and finding the right numbers that work for you will take some practice. But if you give it some time, your routine will start to feel great! Before you know it, you'll be getting some of your best sets and reps, and all that will be happening while others are barely awake, trying to start their day!

CHAPTER 13

CARDIO

"Don't run to add days to your life, run to add life to your days."
—RONALD ROOK

WHEN IT COMES TO GETTING YOUR MORNING WORKOUT EDGE, CARDIO IS another great form of exercise you can add to your daily routine.

For starters, let's clarify that you don't have to run for an hour to improve cardiovascular health and endurance, or (most importantly) to gain your morning workout edge! As a matter of fact, too much cardio can come with diminishing returns for both your health and energy levels. For instance, in a large-scale 2015 study that was published in the *Journal of the American College of Cardiology*, light and moderate joggers were less likely to die than non-runners during the study's two-year follow-up. It is also worth noting that in the same study, strenuous joggers had the same mortality rate as sedentary folks!

In the end, it all comes down to oxidative stress—the physiological damage placed on the body's cells during exercise. Oxidative stress is what spurs the body to recover, grow back stronger and—over time—become healthier. However, when stress levels become too great, the immune system can't keep up. Any form of exercise, when practiced in excess, can contribute to harmful levels of inflammation in the body and also be counterproductive for both mood- and energy-boosting benefits such as the ones we talked about in part one.

So, the right question to ask ourselves here is "what's the minimum effective dose of cardio for our morning workout edge?" Well, there is probably no way to identify one optimal point for everyone. Each person responds to cardiovascular exercise differently based on factors such as overall daily life stressors, genetics, nutrition, and the overall amount of exercise we get per week. When it comes to the old ticker, for example, one hundred and fifty minutes of moderate-intensity exercise (steady-state cardio) per week or seventy-five minutes of vigorous exercise (high-intensity interval training) per week seem to be optimal for cardiovascular health.

In summary, if we were to simplify things and all you do is cardio, thirty minutes each morning (at least five days a week) ensures that you're getting that minimum effective dose, which improves cardiovascular health and endurance but also allows you to maximize your morning workout edge!

Do You Have to Warm-Up for Cardio?

By itself, cardio is a low-intensity activity, so it doesn't take a lot to prepare your body for it. But that doesn't mean that you should jump right into it, particularly if it causes you any discomfort. Especially if you jog on the typical city pavement, I recommend you take a couple of minutes to prepare the body, even if that means that you run a few minutes less.

Now, if you have the extra eleven minutes, I recommend that you start as usual with my morning warm-up routine from Chapter 11 and follow it with the tips below. If you need something faster, try the tips below. Remember, it's better to invest some of your morning workout time in a proper warm-up and get less cardio than doing the opposite.

Here are some tips that will make your morning runs feel smoother while also helping you stay away from injury.

TIP #1: NMS WAKE UP (FOOT ROLLING)

The soles of our feet are extremely sensitive due to their high concentration of nerve endings. This is why massaging your foot is the best way to wake up the NMS (Neuromuscular System) before a cardio activity that has a high impact on your feet. Like most people, if you wear shoes and stand for a couple of hours a day, you will carry a lot of tension in this area. Some even postulate that massaging the bottom of the foot also improves flexibility in the posterior chain, particularly improving flexibility in the hamstrings and the spine (Grieve et al. 2015).

I recommend a minute of foot-rolling per foot. You can start with a tennis ball if you have sensitive feet, but if you want to get some serious work done, I highly recommend you progress to a lacrosse ball. These are pretty inexpensive, and you can find them in most sports stores, both online and off. If this is something you've never tried, there are plenty of tutorials if you do a quick Google search, and I'll also include a link to a personal video at the end of the book. You can even add this to your BSR if you want to save time.

TIP #2: STRETCH THE TIGHT STUFF

You also want to do some light static stretching if you have areas that tend to feel tight during your morning cardio sessions. For most people, these will usually be areas such as the Achilles heel, the hip flexors, and the hamstrings. I recommend thirty seconds of light stretching per area, and all this can be done in less than four minutes.

TIP #3: EASE INTO IT

This is common sense, but I still have to mention it since I've seen people start their morning workouts a lot more aggressively than they should. Besides your muscles and joints, your heart also needs some time to ease into a morning workout, especially a cardiovascular one. So, start with at least ten minutes of the slowest and most low-impact pace possible. For example, jog or even power-walk for ten minutes if you're about to run (or do half and half—five minutes of power-walking and five minutes of very light jogging). If you're about to cycle, pedal on a very light gear first. If you're about to front-crawl swim, first breast-stroke for a few laps. After those ten minutes, very gradually start picking up your regular pace.

CHAPTER 14

HIIT & SPRINTS

"You never beat the hill, but you do get better."
—WALTER PAYTON

SPRINTS AND HIIT ARE FUN TO DO, AND THEY BURN THE SAME NUMBER OF calories in about half the time cardio training does. Some studies have also shown that sprinting increases testosterone and growth hormone levels in young and middle-aged men. These natural anabolic hormones increase strength and muscle growth, and they help you stay lean. They can also increase confidence and sex drive! Overall, they are import-ant for keeping you healthy and vibrant. Short distances and varying speeds are also one of the best ways to train your cardiovascular system. In a way, they are like push-ups for the heart, since they improve cardiovascular function by increasing the amount of blood it can pump!

HIIT (High-Intensity-Interval-Training) and Sprints also leave you with a feeling of serenity. Especially when done outdoors, they produce an amazing mood boost that almost feels like a natural soft drug high. Other than the extra oxygen in your body, the primary suspects for sensa-tions are endorphins and endocannabinoids.

Picking the Right Surface

Over time, running on soft surfaces (e.g., grass) rather than running on hard surfaces (e.g., cement) can make a big difference for your body's joints and connective tissues—the softer the surface, the lower the impact. Because everything in our body is connected, from your foot to your ankle to your knee, and basically all the way up to your cervical spine, the stress and impact of pressure from your feet striking hard ground can cause all kinds of problems in the long run if you're not careful. Ideally, find soft surfaces such as dirt or grass. The best option, in my opinion, especially if you can't run on dirt or grass, is hill sprints!

The Benefits of Running Uphill

As a matter of fact, running uphill was the only way I could teach myself to run again after I got a prosthetic leg. Learning to run on a prosthesis can cause a lot of discomfort at first. In my case, running on a flat surface without any pain initially seemed impossible. But that's when I discovered that short intervals of running uphill was a form of running that caused a much milder impact on my stump.

Even so, I started half-jogging and half-limping in the beginning. Fast forward a couple of years later, and I can nowadays outrun most people my age and younger if we sprint up a hill! No, I'm not saying this in order to brag; it's simply the story behind why I'm so fond of sprints and how I know that they're one of the least-impactful forms of HIIT and sprinting. Well, okay, maybe I also wanted to brag a bit, as well!

Running uphill minimizes the distance your foot has to fall before hitting the ground, therefore creating a lot less impact for your body. Hill sprints are so much more joint-friendly that I'd rather do them on cement than do flat-ground sprints on dirt or grass or even tartan (the professional artificial surface used in track and field stadiums).

Other Benefits of Sprints and HIIT

Especially when done uphill, sprints and HIIT cause your legs to work hard enough to create muscular adaptations similar to those obtained from lifting weights. This makes them a great option for building strong, athletic, and muscular legs if you're more into bodyweight training and calisthenics. Besides training your lower body, they also activate the abdominals, which have to stabilize the pelvis as your legs propel the body forward!

The ideal frequency for HIIT and sprints is two times a week; therefore, I recommend mixing them up with some strength training during the rest of the week.

Finally, I don't know if it's just me, but the hill you sprint on becomes a whole different place. Each time you pass by it, there is a mixed feeling of appreciation, humbleness, intimidation, and respect towards it. The hill is where your legs run uphill and where your soul runs free. It's where you cast your demons. Where you take a load off your heart even though it might feel that it's pounding out of your chest.

Respect the hill!

Warming Up for HIIT and Sprints

Although they target mostly the lower body, there's not a part of your body that is not engaged when performing a sprint workout. This is why I recommend including my eleven-minute morning warm-up routine at the beginning of hill-sprint workouts.

Next, taking your time to get plenty of warm-up rounds is essential. I like to call these warm-up rounds "rehearsal sprints." When it comes to duration, I wouldn't recommend anything shorter than thirty seconds at a high speed if you want to minimize risk of injury. The shorter the sprint after that, the higher the chance of muscle strain.

For example, the hamstring tear is the most common injury I see when people don't take their warm-up seriously before morning sprints and HIIT. Whether you do this type of training in the morning or the afternoon, it's important to realize that in terms of time, the warm-up is more than half the workout! This is why professional sprinters need more than an hour to run one sprint at full capacity!

Since there are a lot of different training approaches in this area as well, I'll once again give you a personal workout example you can adjust and apply to your training. So, let's take hill sprints, which are my favorite sprint workout. Since your body needs a lot of preparation before it's ready to run at a high speed in the morning, you want to start with a couple of rehearsal sets that build the intensity up gradually. Specifically, I recommend at least five rehearsal sets before you start to put in some serious intensity. If you're training in low temperatures, go for a minimum of six rehearsal sets.

To keep things simple and avoid technical terminology that requires calculations and special equipment, I'll use simple cues to give you an estimate of the intensity you want to use. So, here's an example of how my trainees and I warm up prior to a morning hill sprint workout.

REHEARSAL SPRINT ONE AND TWO: ONE MINUTE AT 50 PERCENT

For our first set, we want to run for a minute at fifty percent intensity. An easy way to explain this is using a pace that would allow us to chat with someone or sing without running out of breath. Basically, your first set resembles jogging more than it resembles sprinting.

REHEARSAL SETS THREE AND FOUR: FORTY SECONDS AT 70 PERCENT

For our third round, we're aiming for forty seconds at a pace that wouldn't allow us to chat or sing without running out of breath, but we're still far away from running at high intensity.

REHEARSAL SETS FIVE AND SIX: TWENTY SECONDS AT 80 PERCENT

For our fifth and sixth rounds, we want to slowly start simulating our sprinting pace. Aim for a quick start during the first five seconds, and use a slightly faster pace compared to your previous rehearsal sprints during the middle. Finish off strong again during the last five seconds, using a speed similar to how you'd run during your regular sprints.

Personally, after six rehearsal rounds like these, I'll do two to three thirty-second sprints maximum and complete the workout. If you follow the warm-up to the letter, you won't need more than that to get your morning workout edge! This is also one of my favorite anti-stress workouts!

Overall, experiment with the guidelines above, but always listen to your body and adjust your warm-up rounds accordingly. Never rush through a HIIT or sprint workout in the morning. Give both your heart and the rest of your body time to build up intensity gradually, and always try to sprint smoothly, prioritizing technique over speed.

CHAPTER 15

ALTERNATIVE MORNING CALISTHENICS ROUTINES

"Sometimes you don't have to work hard, you just have to work smart."

—OLD GREEK PROVERB

BASED ON THE TRAINING GUIDELINES PROVIDED SO FAR, YOUR WORKOUTS should take on average thirty to thirty-five minutes, including the warm-up.

If you want something even shorter than that, you can check out the workouts I'll be sharing with you in this extra chapter, since they are my top two favorite shortest and also most effective calisthenics workouts. They don't take more than twelve minutes each (so, combined with my warm-up routine, you can be done in twenty-three minutes!).

These are personally-designed workouts that I use when I have very little time at my disposal (e.g., when I have to go in earlier to work). Since these workouts focus only on the upper body, I like to alternate them with lower-body training days such as hill or stair sprints!

For detailed video tutorials of these workouts, and for more free alternative morning workout routines like these, make sure you have a look again at www.the7AMworkoutedge.com.

Ladder-Based Routines

In a previous chapter, I gave you a general idea of how to structure your morning strength workouts. Still, as I mentioned, there are all kinds of different training approaches and ways to do this.

For example, one of my favorite ways to strength train in the morning is with ladder-based calisthenics routines. For those not familiar with what ladders are, I'll be offering a detailed explanation soon, but for now, here's what you want to keep in mind.

Ladder-based workouts have one of the lowest injury rates when it comes to strength-training, since they build up reps and intensity gradually. In a way, they have an extra warm-up incorporated within the workout! Ladders can build both muscle and strength because they use a broad rep range and stimulate a lot of metabolic stress (what gives you that burning feeling while doing the last rep of a long and tiring set).

Finally, the ladder-based workouts that I'll be sharing with you require one hundred percent of your focus and effort, since they are very efficient at "squeezing in" a lot of training volume and intensity within a very short session. No matter how tight your mornings are on some days, there is always time for a calisthenics ladder workout, especially if you master the following two!

ALTERNATIVE WORKOUT #1: CALISTHENICS SUPER-LADDERS

A super-ladder combines characteristics from both superset and ladder training (ergo the name). For starters, let's define what these terms mean in case you're not familiar with them.

SUPERSETS

A superset is a set of two exercises done back-to-back with no rest in between. This way, you can effectively almost double the amount of work you put into your session, since your resting periods can stay the same. When it comes to calisthenics, you can use supersets to either target the same main movement pattern or even antagonist movement patterns. In this case, though, we'll be targeting one common main movement pattern per super-ladder.

LADDERS

A traditional ladder focuses on doing one exercise at a time, using a series of sets done with an ascending and descending repetition pattern.

For example, let's say we do a pull-up ladder. This means that you typically start by doing one pull-up and you rest for a short amount of time. Next, you do two pull-ups, and you rest again for the same short amount of time. Next, you do three pull-ups, and so on, until you reach technical failure (the point you can't do another rep with proper form).

Now, let's say you reach technical failure once you get in eight pull-ups. After this point, you have to also *go down the ladder* again in the same fashion. Therefore, your next set is seven pull-ups followed by a short resting period, six pull-ups followed again by the same short resting period, etc., until you once again reach a single rep.

Especially when it comes to morning workouts, I recommend going up and down ladders either one or two reps at a time.

SUPER-LADDER

Finally, a super-ladder is a ladder where, instead of doing one exercise, you superset (combine without rest in between) two exercises that belong to the same movement pattern, either a pull or a push. So, during each superset, you start with the most challenging exercise and follow it with double the reps for the second exercise, taking twenty-one seconds of rest between each superset (if this is not clear yet, keep reading, and it will make sense soon).

You keep adding reps in the same fashion until you reach technical failure, which we'll call the top of the ladder. Once you reach the top of the ladder, you take one to two minutes of rest, and after your resting period is over, you go down the ladder again in the same fashion.

SUPER-LADDER EXAMPLES

Let's say you pick chest dips and push-ups for your calisthenics Push Super-Ladder. And let's also assume that you can go up the ladder until you reach technical failure at five chest-dips and ten push-ups.

Here's how this would look:

- Superset #1: **one dip** followed by **two push-ups** and twenty-one seconds of rest

- Superset #2: **two dips** followed by **four push-ups** and twenty-one seconds of rest

- Superset #3: **three dips** followed by **six push-ups** and twenty-one seconds of rest

- Superset #4: **four dips** followed by **eight push-ups** and twenty-one seconds of rest

- Superset #5: **five dips** followed by **ten push-ups** and twenty-one seconds of rest

Rest for one to two minutes.

- Superset #6: **four dips** followed by **eight push-ups** and twenty-one seconds of rest

- Superset #7: **three dips** followed by **six push-ups** and twenty-one seconds of rest

- Superset #8: **two dips** followed by **four push-ups** and twenty-one seconds of rest

- Superset #9: **one dip** followed by **two push-ups** and twenty-one seconds of rest

Here are a few more calisthenics options that work great:

- If you want a more advanced calisthenics push super-ladder, you can superset handstand push-ups with dips.

- For something more intermediate, other than chest dips followed by push-ups, you can also superset pike push-ups with regular push-ups.

- Finally, for a more beginner calisthenics super-ladder, I recommend regular or incline push-ups followed by bodyweight tricep extensions.

The same goes for pull super-ladders. Some of my favorite calisthenics super-ladder exercises are the following:

- Pull-ups followed by chin-ups (don't double the reps for the second exercise in this case, since chin-ups are only slightly easier than pull-ups)

- Pull-ups followed by inverted rows (this is usually the most popular choice among my trainees)

- Band-assisted pull-ups followed by incline inverted rows (ideal for beginners)

By the way, if you want to include both a push and a pull super-ladder in one workout, I recommend that you start with the push super-ladder first and take at least five minutes of rest in between to make sure you have enough strength to conquer the pull super-ladder next.

ALTERNATIVE WORKOUT #2: CALISTHENICS DROP-LADDERS

Drop-ladders are a bit similar to super-ladders, and they combine characteristics from both drop-set and ladder training.

WHAT ARE CALISTHENIC DROP SETS?

During a traditional weight-lifting drop set, you start by focusing on completing a set until failure. You then lighten the load and repeat with little to no rest in between sets. Since when it comes to calisthenics the only load available is usually your own bodyweight, I like to practice what I call calisthenic drop sets, in the following way:

First of all, instead of focusing on a single exercise, you focus on a movement pattern, starting with one of the most challenging exercises that belongs to that movement pattern. After that, the way you drop the intensity during the next set is by switching to an easier exercise that belongs to the same movement pattern.

For example:

- If you start with a pull-up, you can next switch to an inverted row or a chin-up.

- If you start with whole bodyweight rows, you can switch to basic inverted rows.

- If you start with a chest dip, you can move to a push-up.

- If you start with a single leg wall-sit, you can progress to a bilateral wall-sit.

You can use drop-ladders to train one movement pattern, or you can even combine them to train the whole body in one session, as I'll be showing you in the example below.

DROP-LADDER ROUTINE

Let's say we use chest dips and push-ups for our example. Since you always begin with the most challenging exercise of the two, start with chest dips and go up the ladder, one or two reps at a time with twenty-one seconds of rest in between each set. At the top of the ladder, take two minutes of rest.

If you reach technical failure at ten chest dips, this is how it will look:

- Two chest-dips followed by twenty-one seconds of rest

- Four chest dips followed by twenty-one seconds of rest

- Six chest dips followed by twenty-one seconds of rest

- Eight chest dips followed by twenty-one seconds of rest

- Ten chest dips followed by twenty-one seconds of rest

When it comes to drop-ladders, we only do half a ladder, meaning you only climb up to the top and you don't go back down again. Therefore, once we reach technical failure on the way up, after our two minutes of rest, we then move on to our push-up ladder—this time, though, starting at the rep range we failed during our previous, more challenging exercise!

So, let's say we reach technical failure for our push-up ladder at sixteen reps. Here's how it will look:

- Ten push-ups followed by twenty-one seconds of rest

- Twelve push-ups followed by twenty-one seconds of rest

- Fourteen push-ups followed by twenty-one seconds of rest

- Sixteen push-ups followed by twenty-one seconds of rest

Once you reach this point, your workout is over!

PART 4

MORNING NUTRITION

INTRODUCTION

Ah, nutrition: definitely the most complicated, debatable, and unresolved subject when it comes to fitness and health. The reason that nutrition can be so diverse is that people simply differ.

For example, genetics, biological quirks, and physiological anomalies can affect what works best for everyone. Just as no two people have matching fingerprints, neither do they have identical biochemical characteristics. We have different digestive, absorptive, and enzymatic patterns, and therefore different nutrient needs. This is why there is no average diet that will fit everyone's biochemical individuality perfectly. If one person's body differs even by an increment in how it digests, absorbs, and excretes one mineral over a day, think of the difference that can make over a period of weeks or months. As a result, this person may require significantly more of a specific nutrient to stay healthy.

Besides differing on a physiological level, we also have different lifestyles, and we often see things from a different ethical standpoint, which can also affect our nutritional choices. In summary, you can't give a hundred people the same nutritional plan (as healthy as it might seem) and expect all hundred people to thrive. It's important to learn to observe how your body reacts to different dietary approaches and see what works best for you. For example, some people do great on more vegetarian-oriented diets, while others thrive on more ketogenic (protein-based) diets.

This is why even though I do offer nutritional strategies, I never offer canned diet plans to the general public (e.g., eat X grams of chicken with X grams of brown rice for dinner), especially through books or the internet! An effective nutritional plan should always be a hundred percent personalized.

Breakfast: Not Necessarily the Most Important Meal of the Day

For decades, the common notion was that the moment you wake up, your body needs a meal (typically rich in carbs) in order to have energy and start the day properly. Especially during the last fifteen years, though, this has changed. Not eating at the start of the day or even for hours after that (what is also called intermittent fasting), has become a popular approach a lot of people follow.

Prepackaged and ready-to-eat breakfast cereals began with the American temperance movement in the nineteenth century, which is quite a small segment of time for a species that has been around for thousands of years. Think about it from an evolutionary standpoint. Our hunter and gatherer ancestors who lived in the wild would not always have food available to them the moment they woke up. It makes sense, therefore, that not everyone's body should be that fragile when it comes to skipping breakfast.

In the 1830s, the Reverend Sylvester Graham preached the virtues of a vegetarian diet to his congregation—and, in particular, the importance of whole-meal flour. "Meat-eating," he said, "excited the carnal passions." After that, the Seventh-Day Adventists John Harvey Kellogg took up the mission. He set about devising cures for what he believed were the common ills of the day: in particular, constipation and masturbation. Disturbing, right? Still, in Kellogg's mind, the two were closely linked, so he started producing an easily-digested form of cereal.

Slowly, somewhere around the beginning of the twentieth century, we were convinced that we needed perfectly shaped rings or puffy flakes from a colorful and beautifully marketed box to start the day.

That's right: breakfast cereal was a trend set by religious fundamentalists!

To Eat or Not to Eat?

In most healthy individuals, cortisol levels rise sharply for approximately thirty minutes after awakening. By sixty minutes, they usually reach their peak. This normal spike of cortisol helps break down body fat by increasing the release of fatty acids for fuel. Besides our normal spike of cortisol, there is also a release of anabolic hormones that promote muscle growth and maintenance. In a way, our body is smart enough to produce its own breakfast by tapping into our fat reserves and keeping muscle tissue intact. By the way, the reason I'm mentioning muscle tissue here is because some used to fear that training on an empty stomach in the morning might break down muscle.

In summary, if you've had a decent dinner the previous day, and you keep your morning workout short (as recommended in this book), you can easily train fasted without worrying about your body cannibalizing its own muscle tissue. And from my experience, when it comes to short 7 A.M. Workout Edge type of workouts, a lot of people perform better when they train fasted. I have done my best workouts during a fasted state. Now, does everybody have to train fasted? Of course not!

Although a lot of people (including me) feel better by skipping breakfast and even perform better during their morning workout, this isn't the case for everyone. There are plenty of other people that feel as if they might not make it through the workout alive if they train on an empty stomach.

Overall, I find that when it comes to morning exercise and nutrition, there are two main categories of people:

1. Those who need at least a little something before the workout (whom, for simplicity, we'll call "the non-fasting 7 A.M.-ers")

2. Those for whom training fasted works a lot better, whom we'll call "the fasting 7 A.M.ers"

In general, if training fasted works for you, that's great. All you need is to get some fluids (water, tea, coffee, etc.) in you during your BSR and you'll do just fine. If you're the first type though, you need to set up a proper pre-workout snack.

CHAPTER 16

THE NON-FASTING 7 A.M.-ER

"To eat is a necessity, but to eat intelligently is an art."
—FRANÇOIS DE ROCHEFOUCAULD

IF YOU BELONG TO THIS CATEGORY OF PEOPLE, YOU'LL NEED TO SET UP A pre-workout snack that will give you some fuel but can also be metabolized and digested quickly. I recommend incorporating this at the beginning of your BSR so you workout twenty to thirty minutes after you eat.

Pre-Workout Snack Structure

As we said, everyone is different, but usually the following formula works best:

- *50 percent simple carbs:* you need a source of fuel that will be quickly accessible to your muscles

- *30 to 40 percent fat:* fat digests slower, and a little bit of it before you train will help curb your morning hunger and provide you with a more stable stream of energy across the workout

- *10 to 20 percent protein:* protein will also help curb
  your morning hunger, and when broken down, it
  will provide amino acids to aid your muscles later on

SIMPLE CARBS

Complex carbs are usually less processed, and they are typically considered a healthier choice, whereas simple carbs
have a bad reputation. This does not mean that all simple
carbs are bad, though. Simple carbs occur naturally in some
foods that can be part of a balanced diet—and, in our case,
they're what we need in a pre-workout meal that will fuel
us shortly before training.

Simple carbs are the quickest-burning fuel, since they can
quickly provide your bloodstream with sugar molecules—
not a bad thing if you're about to make good use of them
by working out within the coming half-hour.

A great simple carb source, for example, can be fruit. Not
all fruits will do, though. You want to avoid citrus fruits, since
they tend to cause problems on an empty stomach, especially
when it comes to gastroesophageal reflux issues. Instead, go
for the sweeter fruits that sit well on your stomach and digest
better in the morning. For most people, these will be fruits
like apples, bananas, peaches, melons, pears, watermelon,
raspberries, grapes, blackberries, blueberries, kiwi, etc.

If you're not a fan of fruits in the morning, you can also
spread your healthy fats on a rice cake, which will provide
you with some quickly digestible carbs and will be digested
quickly. More on this soon.

FATS

As to fats, nut spreads are the most practical solution; plus, they are decent protein and mineral sources. Keep in mind that some brands are packed with sugar, so try to go the healthier route by purchasing all-natural nut spreads. You can even make your own. To most people, nut spreads taste great when combined with sweet fruits. Peanut butter and almond butter are some typical popular choices here.

PEANUT BUTTER VERSUS ALMOND BUTTER

Almond butter is slightly more nutritious than peanut butter in terms of vitamins, minerals, and fiber; but peanut butter has a little more protein than almond butter. Both nut butters are roughly equal in calories and sugar. Overall, you can say they're equally healthy, so it just comes down to personal taste.

NUT BUTTER ALTERNATIVE?

If you are allergic to nuts, you can also consider seed spreads. You may be able to consume seeds because none of them are tree nuts. Not only are seed spreads a good alternative, but tahini is my top choice when it comes to healthy morning fats.

Still, especially if you are prone to food allergies, you should always consult a specialist before trying something you've never had before.

WHAT THE FRACK IS TAHINI?

Although a staple of Mediterranean cuisine, a lot of people are not familiar with tahini. Tahini is a paste made from sesame seeds. It typically has a smooth texture similar to nut butter but a stronger and more savory taste that's often described as bitter. It is relatively low in calories (thirty calories per teaspoon) but high in fiber, protein, and an assortment of essential vitamins and minerals (copper, selenium, phosphorus, iron, zinc, and calcium).

In addition to providing a wealth of nutrients, tahini also has been associated with several health benefits, including improved heart health, reduced inflammation, and potential cancer-fighting effects.

HOW MUCH?

Keep your snack between one hundred and two hundred calories. Stay more on the low end if you're a smaller guy or a woman. If you're a guy and you have a big build, go for the higher end.

Here are some numbers for you to keep in mind:

- One medium-sized banana is 100 calories.

- A teaspoon of almond or peanut butter is fifty calories (it's actually thirty-five, but I know you like to fill that teaspoon a bit more... Am I wrong?).

- One rice cake is usually around thirty-five calories.

EXAMPLES

Based on the above numbers, here are some examples of pre-workout snacks for the non-fasting 7 A.M.-er:

- *150 calories:* one medium-sized banana with a teaspoon of almond butter

- *100 calories:* one apple with one teaspoon of peanut butter

- *200 calories:* one rice cake with one large-sized banana and one teaspoon of tahini

Keep in mind that these are mostly ideas to get you started. Think of them as a template you can slowly adjust and refine based on your nutritional preferences and what you believe best fits your own biochemical individuality.

CHAPTER 17

POST-MORNING WORKOUT NUTRITION

"Exercise is king. Nutrition is queen. Put them together and you've got a kingdom."
—JACK LALANNE

Your post-workout meal (what most people would call breakfast)—if you decide to have it, that is—will be your first meal of the day. I say this even for those of you non-fasting 7 A.M.-ers, since what you have pre-workout is more of a snack than a meal.

I believe the first main meal of the day determines the nutritional tone of the rest of the day, so no matter what time you have it, or how big or small it is, make it a good one! No, I don't mean filling up a bowl with refined carbohydrates and sugar that come from that huge colorful box marketed as healthy by advertisement companies. Nor am I talking about toaster pastries, doughnuts, or any of that processed stuff filled with sugar which a big number of people call breakfast.

If that's what you consider breakfast, it's time to make some changes. This is not how you want to start the day, and it is definitely not how you want to fuel your body after a morning workout.

What Is a Healthy Breakfast?

What you want to focus on mostly are non-processed whole foods. Things such as organic eggs and quality oatmeal. Real, thick, creamy fatty yogurt, like authentic Greek yogurt (not that fake white gelatinous watered-down version that is often passed off to you as yogurt). If you want something faster, you can also make yourself a nice, healthy smoothie.

If you want some juice, avoid the boxed stuff; get some oranges and grapefruits instead, and squeeze yourself some fresh juice! It's not so difficult, and you probably already know what you should be eating, after all: real, healthy food that is minimally processed and ideally cooked by you! It's not hard; it simply needs some preparation and getting organized.

Next, you also want to choose foods that sit well on your stomach. What might be a great option for me might not be ideal for you—even if it's considered a healthy choice! When your body digests food fast and feels energetic afterwards instead of lethargic, that is usually one more sign that what you're eating fits your biochemical individuality best. So, find foods that do not irritate your stomach or feel like a struggle to digest.

Especially in the beginning of the day, you don't want things that weigh you down and make you want to crawl back in bed to sleep it off. Of course, that's not just a matter of quality; it's also about quantity. Overeating anything can throw your energy off.

Ideally, you want something that has some easily digestible protein, carbs, and a bit of healthy fat.

Here are some ideas:

- Eggs

- Nuts

- Leafy veggies

- Tomatoes

- Fruit

- Oatmeal

- Cottage cheese

- Yogurt

- Homemade whole wheat bread

- Sourdough bread

- Real butter

Simplicity and Specificity Beat Complexity

Simplicity and specificity beat complexity… This is a motto I live by, especially when it comes to nutrition! Monday through Saturday, 99 percent of my post-workout meals during the last five years have been the same thing.

Yes, I do have whatever I feel like on Sundays, with pancakes being at the top of my list—but here's what I eat during the other mornings of the week, without even the slightest deviation:

- Three eggs (boiled or fried)

- Two hundred grams of cottage cheese

- Two thin slices of toasted whole wheat bread

- A portion or two of fruit or veggies that are ideally in season

I know, it's not something anyone today would consider social-media worthy! When I tell this to people, a lot of them find me insanely boring and even weird. But there's a reason behind this!

First of all, it takes me less than five minutes to prepare this meal. Second of all, it helps me hit my protein target by the end of the day, which I consider highly important for satiety (protein is the most satiating micronutrient) and my muscle-building and maintenance goals. And last, combined with the rest of my day's meals, it also gives me all the rest of the nutrients I need.

If you're still wondering how I don't find this boring, day in and day out—well, personally, I find that when I feel like eating after a fasted morning workout, I don't need variety or a special meal to get my appetite going! I'm almost always hungry, and that is why this simple meal tastes amazing every time! Trust me, if I had to spend an hour preparing those flashy types of breakfasts you see on influencer social media feeds, I'd rather go back to eating donuts or cereal!

But that's how I am. In the morning, I need to be quick and efficient, as I imagine a lot of you reading this book also have to be. Sure, you don't have to be as extreme and minimal as I am, and you can have two or three typical breakfast recipes on rotation to keep things more interesting. Hey, you can even make a different influencer photo-worthy kind of breakfast every day if you don't mind everything that goes with it (all the extra time preparing, doing complex grocery shopping, etc.). If that's something you enjoy, go for it!

But, whatever you choose to do, make sure it's realistic and practical in the long run. As I said, this is not a recipe or diet book. I have given you an approach to follow here, so the next step is to simply experiment and figure out what works for you! If you want something more specific, I prefer giving you the following advice rather than giving you canned examples that might work for some but not at all for others.

My advice is: hire a proper nutritionist! Once you have a specialist help you figure out the best options for you, even though it might cost you some extra bucks, you've made an investment that will pay off—you'll have something custom-tailored that you can use for the rest of your life.

PART 5

STAYING ON TRACK

INTRODUCTION

After being on track with my morning routine and experiencing the 7 A.M. Workout Edge's effect on my life, something unexpected happened. The world as we knew it suddenly changed due to a pandemic caused by…well, unless you're reading this book in the far distant future, you know I'm talking about Covid-19. A virus that kept us locked up at home, disrupted our daily routine, and turned out to stay for a lot longer than we originally estimated.

This was the first time I fell off the wagon with my 7 A.M. Workout Edge. After months of not having missed a single workout, a few weeks into my first lockdown, I found my routine breaking down. It's kind of ironic when you think about it, since I created this routine initially as a solution to making sure I stayed consistent with my training while having a hectic work and life schedule. And yet, I ended up getting side-tracked because the opposite occurred—I now had more time than ever!

So, why did this happen, then? Well, here's how it started…

Seeing that I had the extra time while working from home, I thought to myself, "I can finally get some extra sleep without stressing about getting up early in the morning." But, with each hour that I postponed my morning workout, my motivation to exercise decreased. It turns out that laziness just breeds more laziness! Like so many of us during the quarantines, I found myself overanalyzing every action and extra activity that I could now incorporate into my daily routine, only to end up doing fewer things.

It turns out that more time doesn't always equal more productivity or motivation. As I mentioned in the beginning of the book, it is human nature to stay motivated just enough to only get things done that cover our primal needs. Once those needs are covered, our mind always looks for the path of least resistance and most procrastination! So, the more time you have, the more you look for distractions and reasons to do less.

CHAPTER 18

HOW I USED THE 7 A.M. WORKOUT EDGE TO CUT THROUGH THE QUARANTINE SLUMP

"A mistake repeated more than once is a decision."
—PAULO COELHO

PRIOR TO COVID-19, MANY OF US WOULD OFTEN WISH TO HAVE MORE FREE time to get better at the guitar, to learn a new language, to cook, or to do this and do that. Yet, how many people do you know who followed through with these wishes when we were gifted all that free time during the Covid-19 lockdowns?

From what I saw in my circle of people, very few!

The reason so many of us fell into a slump wasn't the virus or the lockdowns. It was our reaction to it. It was our belief that we can be productive and proactive without any structure. But, instead of doing all the things we'd always dreamed of doing if we had more free time, we simply woke up later in the day, and we kept postponing our to-do list and all the new stuff we'd start doing.

We'd spend most of the day in the same sweatpants we slept in, drinking coffee, binge eating, watching TV shows, and eating less healthy foods (although we finally had time to cook more healthy foods). Before we knew it, it would be dark outside. Another day would be gone, and we'd tell ourselves we'd do things differently tomorrow. Well, at least that was how my first week went by. Until all this started to look familiar.

The pandemic had a lot of similarities to my accident. They were both unexpected, and they had me closed up at home for large amounts of time. And even though I was healthy and mobile this time, I felt the temptation to stay in bed again due to all the mental implications so many of us experienced during the lockdowns and quarantines.

COVID-19 reminded me that life won't always flow the way you want it to flow. Things will often be stale when you want them to move faster, and they'll be hectic when you want them to move slower. Occasionally, you'll have periods when everything will be clicking and going your way, but more often than not, you'll have turbulence and obstacles on your path.

Having spent the last years building my local personal coaching practice, only to have the lockdowns begin the moment things started to really take off for my business wasn't pleasant. I was actually quite pissed off that I couldn't work, and I felt tempted to blame the situation instead of being proactive and figuring out alternatives. It is always easier to victimize yourself when things seem out of control.

But, I decided I wasn't going to make that mistake twice in my life! Having wasted all those years after my accident in the same way once was enough. So, I snapped out of the pandemic funk, and I got back to getting things done! I used my morning workout edge to clear my head, begin my morning with confidence, and build momentum to help me stay productive during the rest of the day.

The 7 A.M. Workout Edge helped me stay in charge of my days during COVID-19. It helped me make the conscious decision to see those years as an opportunity, instead of an obstacle. I could finally make up for so much of the lost time and do all the things I had been wanting to do for years but never managed due to time restrictions!

Things such as:

- Reading all the books I had been postponing the last couple of years.

- Learning to play the piano.

- Improving the online part of the business.

- Studying cinematography and story-telling in order to improve my YouTube channel.

- Minimizing social media usage to use my time even more intentionally.

- Adopting a more minimalist lifestyle by getting rid of things that didn't have any importance in my life, donating clothes, and simplifying my living space and wardrobe.

- Doing a lot of self-work and figuring out the kind of person I want to be and the life I want to live.

And, finally, this was when I created an online course called the 7 A.M. Workout Club, where I tested and validated all the main principles from this book. After the course was a success, I got serious about completing this book, which was another thing I had been delaying for a while!

CHAPTER 19

NEVER MISS TWICE

"What starts as an excuse can easily become a habit. Don't let a bad day become a lifestyle."
—JAMES CLEAR

THE WAY I FELL INTO A SLUMP DURING THE FIRST LOCKDOWN STARTED WITH ONE missed workout. Even though I had been on a roll with my morning workout edge for months, and even though my morning routine had become something sacred to me, suddenly missing one session due to our lives being turned upside down by Covid-19 threw me completely off my game. No, it wasn't the main reason, but that first missed session triggered a domino effect of more and more missed workouts that threw me into a slump.

A lot of people have had this experience while starting a workout routine. It typically looks something like this:

Things are going great, and you're on track for a while. You're feeling excited! You're making progress, and sticking to the routine feels doable, until…one day, you miss one session. Suddenly, you feel your momentum is gone. For some reason, that one missed session, after being on a streak for so long, has a very negative impact on your motivation. You start to doubt yourself, and pessimistic thoughts from the past creep into your head. Maybe they sound something like this: "I guess I'm just not the disciplined workout type of person." Or something like this: "I guess that was it. I gave it my best shot, but I just find working out boring." And you keep falling into that dark rabbit hole.

Before you know it, that one missed day has turned into a week. After a month, you're on the couch eating take-out, watching Netflix or playing video games, and you're wondering why you have zero willpower to get started again. If not with exercise, we've all experienced this in the past when trying to build a new habit, whether with a diet we want to follow, learning to play a musical instrument, writing a book, learning a new language, or working on a side-business, etc.

So, how do you avoid the downward spiral one missed session can cause? How do you rebuild your momentum?

Never Miss Twice

Even if you've already created what feels like an effortless bulletproof morning routine, and your morning workout edge has begun to change your life, you have to keep in mind that life won't always go according to your plans. As perfectly as you schedule your days, hiccups will eventually show up in your programming every now and then. Eventually, we all miss a workout. Yes, even us 7 A.M.-ers! Maybe you'll have to take your kid unexpectedly to the doctor (knock on wood, you won't). Maybe your phone will malfunction, and your alarm clock won't go off. Or maybe you'll just wake up in a really shitty mood. Hey, it happens to all of us; don't sweat it.

The problem is not that one missed workout. The real problem is when a single missed workout triggers a domino effect of more missed workouts. What you want to realize on such occasions is that a common characteristic of people who are consistent with their training routine is not that they never miss workouts; it's that when they do, they rebound quickly! In other words, the problem is not falling off the wagon, but not getting back on it as fast as possible afterwards.

This is why the solution is simple, and it works: stick to the "never miss twice" rule! Instead of taking self-criticizing guilt-trips or feeling disappointed for that one missed workout, forget about it and focus on not missing the next one. Whatever happens, no matter how unmotivated you feel, make that next workout happen! I first read about this rule in James Clear's book *Atomic Habits*, one of my favorite books on habit formation. What the "never miss twice" rule does so successfully is allow you to give yourself a break without falling into a rut. As long as you make the next one, missing one workout every now and then is not a problem. It's just life!

Missing two sessions, though, is the beginning of a pattern. And putting a stop to this before it snowballs towards the opposite direction is crucial. As James Clear says: "What starts as an excuse can easily become a habit. Don't let a bad day become a lifestyle."

As simple as it sounds, the "never miss twice" rule works! In the end, what separates successful people from quitters is that they always get back on their routine, and they never miss twice.

CHAPTER 20

KEEPING TRACK OF YOUR MORNING WORKOUT EDGE

"The best thing about the future is that it comes one day at a time."
—ABRAHAM LINCOLN

ONE OF THE MOST SIMPLE THINGS THAT HELPS PEOPLE TO STICK TO A NEW HABIT is habit tracking. In a nutshell, habit tracking is measuring whether or not you performed your habit on any given day. Usually, it involves marking off a day on a simple calendar (digital or physical), and it works best for things you want to do on a more regular basis (it is not as useful for more sporadic activities like doing your taxes).

I don't believe that measuring a habit is something you have to do in the long run. After all, you already have a ton of habits in your life that run perfectly without you tracking them, since once a habit is firmly established, it becomes more effortless over time. Often, a habit becomes automated to the point that you don't even think about it so much anymore, since it almost runs by itself. It's our brain's way of being more efficient so we can do more things while using fewer cognitive resources.

But, until a set of behaviors that form a habit become habitual—especially when it comes to more complex new habits, like a whole morning routine revolving around morning exercise—keeping track of them during those first few weeks or months can be very helpful.

What Are the Benefits of Habit Tracking?

Using a tracking system while forming a new behavioral pattern can provide a visual record of your habit streak. This way, you have access to visual proof that serves as a reminder of all your hard work and how far you've come, making you think twice before breaking that streak—something that helps reinforce the whole process and empowers you to keep going. Each checkbox becomes a little brick that is building the foundation for something bigger and more rigid each day.

Your habit tracker helps you stay on course, and it reminds you that you're on the right path. This is why it is a good idea to place your tracking system somewhere that will make it noticeable prior to your habit. Seeing more and more of your previous ticked boxes each morning will remind you of your commitment and motivate you to cross off that next box. For example, when it comes to your morning workout routine, print your habit tracker and place it somewhere high-profile, such as next to the coffee machine, on the fridge, or on the bathroom door.

Filling in your habit tracker each day creates a reward system, which is a key part of building habits. Yes, even little things, such as the anticipation of filling in that checkbox once again, help. It might not seem like a lot, but it can make the whole process addictive! Each time you cross a day or tick it on your phone, your brain gets a small dopamine hit, which feeds your desire to continue the habit.

Sure, our morning workout routine will reward us with a lot more than the satisfaction of crossing off one more day in our calendar; but until our new habit builds enough momentum for us to start experiencing the true potential of the morning workout edge, little behavior-forming hacks like habit tracking can be quite helpful!

How to Keep Track

There are many ways to do this, but the more visual your tracking system is, the better. I recommend that you go old-school and simply print a monthly calendar, crossing off each day when you successfully practice your morning routine. If you're more of an app person, there are a ton of apps you can download, as well.

Just search for a habit tracker in your smartphone's app store. Still, my recommendation is that you print your first two months and keep that piece of paper somewhere you can see it first thing in the morning. After that, feel free to go digital.

In the long run, I believe most people can ditch their trackers, since relying on how much more awesome each day feels when you reap the morning workout edge becomes enough of a reminder by itself! Until then, though, and especially during the first six weeks, I highly recommend filling in a daily tracker.

To summarize everything, here's how to get started:

- Step #1: Buy a traditional paper calendar (or print one online).

- Step #2: Place your calendar somewhere that is hard to miss during your morning routine.

- Step #3: Each time you get your morning workout in, cross the day off with a big X.

CHAPTER 21

THE 7 A.M. WORKOUT EDGE BRAIN WIND-DOWN ROUTINE

"The best bed that a man can sleep on is peace."
—SOMALI PROVERB

TECHNOLOGY NOWADAYS HAS INCREASED CHOICES DRAMATICALLY IN BOTH GOOD and bad ways. One of the downsides is that we now always have the choice to be working. The office doors don't close at 5 p.m. anymore. Every minute we spend relaxing is also a minute we could be working. This turns every moment into a decision, and it's something we didn't have to deal with in the past!

Think about it. These days, when you come home, you can still carry your work with you, whether we're talking about your smartphone or laptop. This doesn't mean that you necessarily feel like working all the time, but it is still a conscious decision you have to make. For example, even spending time with your kid can be a decision between actually paying attention to your daughter or answering email! Unless you have a way to draw a line and separate when work ends and leisure time starts, your mind won't be able to fully unwind.

How you end the day affects how you'll start the next morning. If you're all stressed out, your sleep will suffer, and you'll wake up less motivated to do anything the next day. This is why having a wind-down routine can be extremely helpful if you want to make sure you'll fall asleep early and also get quality sleep. And although working out early in the day is one of the best things you can do to improve sleep, if you still find yourself struggling to fall asleep as early as you'd like to, having a strategy to wind down before bed is a must.

If you do a quick google search, you'll find a ton of tips and wind-down routines that are supposed to help you unwind and sleep earlier and better, such as using scented candles, dimming the lights, playing calming music, avoiding screen time before bed, etc. To be honest, although I don't think these hurt, I also don't believe that they make much of a difference.

Having struggled with sleep a lot in the past, I know they don't do a lot when you're seriously wired up, especially for those with bad sleep. There are studies showing that more than half of people in the US lie awake at night due to stress.

In the end, I believe that no matter how much you try to set the ideal sleeping conditions around you, if your mind is not at ease, it doesn't make that much of a difference. This is why we call it "falling asleep"—because you can't force yourself to do it! Rather, you have to be able to let go of stressing about tomorrow and dwelling over today, yesterday, and the days before that.

Easier said than done, right?

Tired but Wired

One of the worst things at the end of a long day is having that "tired but wired" feeling while trying to fall asleep—feeling your body needs rest while having your mind running a hundred miles per hour.

A big reason I find this happens for a lot of people is that although work has ended hours ago, they're mentally still at the office. Often, even though we think work ends once we turn off our screens, start packing up our things, and leave our workspace…our mind can stay in work mode long after all that. This can be even worse for those working from home, since there is no distinct separation between work and personal life.

Of course, other than work, there are a lot of things that can keep us tense and delay our sleep, whether it's stress over our personal life, finances, or even deeper existential rabbit holes! Whatever the case, at the end of the day, when you're tired, lacking clarity, and your mind is prone to falling into anxiety loops, a wind-down routine can be a very valuable tool to help you let go and speed up the falling asleep process.

Setting Up Your Brain Wind-Down Routine (BWR)

No matter what has your mind running a hundred miles per hour, your BWR is meant to help you slow down, until it's time to park yourself in bed and fall asleep as effortlessly as possible. Your BWR should start at least three hours before your preferred sleeping time. During that time, you want to schedule mainly relaxing activities and nothing work related. The best recipe I've found, and have also applied successfully with a lot of other people I personally coach, can be summarized in the following four steps:

1. DAILY REVIEW

The first step for helping yourself to unload and set the process of winding down in motion is a list of all the left-over pending things and loose ends you have for the next day. Storing these in your memory only creates unnecessary cognitive load and stress, especially at the end of a long day. By capturing them on paper or in an app on your phone, you'll be able to let go of them a lot easier instead of having them poking at your mind for hours after work. Ideally, you want to do this at work (or whatever you consider your work environment) and not at home.

2. LOG OUT

Once you're done with your daily review, you want to cut off all channels of communication—digital and other, if possible—with anything and anyone work-related. Do whatever you can to separate your work environment from your home environment, even if you have a home office or you work at home! Lock the office door, shut down your laptop, turn off email notifications, log out from work-related communication networks, etc.

Personally, I like to shut off everything internet-related after this point. Social media platforms, Viber, WhatsApp—every single thing! After all, if there's something urgent, people can reach out to me by calling my personal number.

Steps one and two (daily review and logging out) mean that you might have to spend an extra fifteen minutes taking care of loose ends before you leave work, but being able to detach from your work environment—physically, digitally, and, most importantly, mentally—is crucial for a good night's sleep.

3. MOVE (LIGHT OUTDOOR EXERCISE)

After step two, I recommend some light outdoor exercise. Even a walk around the block before dinner can make a difference! Especially if you work indoors, getting some fresh air before settling down at home is vital. Personally, my wind-down routine is also my book time of the day. Once I'm done at work, I put on my headphones, and I listen to an audiobook while going for a walk. Depending on how wound-up I am, this can be anywhere between twenty minutes and an hour and a half!

If light outdoor exercise is not an option, or not something you're in the mood to do after work (maybe your work already involves plenty of outdoor activity), and you prefer something more static or indoor, some other options I've found helpful over time are mindfulness meditation, stretching routines, and light yoga routines.

4. SUIT OUT

As soon as you can, get out of your work clothes! There's something about having a nice warm shower and wearing something clean, fresh, and comfortable—your pajamas, your favorite couch sweat-pants and t-shirt, or whatever it is that you feel comfortable in.

5. CHILL!

Once you're done with all four of these steps, find something relaxing to do. Things such as cooking, eating, connecting with loved ones, reading a relaxing novel, or any hobby that helps you unwind (e.g., playing some music), or even catching up on a favorite TV show are all perfectly valid options.

What about Screens and Blue Light?

I think that blue light and screen time before bed has been demonized and blown out of proportion. If done in moderation, I believe that for most of us it isn't something that can really harm our sleep. Of course, I do recommend blue light filters and using the lowest brightness setting on any screen (TVs, laptops, tablets, smartphones, etc.) you'll be using once you set your BWR in motion. And sure, I'd rather spend the night under the stars on my balcony or read a paperback, but that's not always practical or something everyone feels like doing at the end of a long day!

If you follow all the previous steps, I seriously doubt that a little bit of screen time will negatively impact your sleep. If you find that watching your favorite show for thirty to sixty minutes relaxes you and helps you fall asleep, forget about the screen haters! Just go ahead and make it part of your BWR. Personally, kicking back for half an hour with a favorite show in bed is one of my most effective final unwinding steps that helps me fall asleep early. Just try to watch something light or funny and not something too intense (thrillers, dramas, etc.)!

In summary, having also personally struggled with sleep a lot in the past, I find that everything always goes back to normal when I stay true to my morning workout and my wind-down routine!

CHAPTER 22

POWER NAPS

"Sleep is the best meditation."
—DALAI LAMA

MEDITERRANEAN PEOPLE LOVE THEIR MIDDAY NAP—OR, AS THE SPANISH CALL it, their siesta. For most Greeks, this means about an hour of sleep during lunch break (which lasts about three hours, since we typically work from 8:30 a.m. to 1:30 p.m., and then from 5:30 to 8:30 p.m.). Although this never was my thing, on the rare occasion that I would accidentally fall asleep midday, I would always feel groggier, sleepier, and unmotivated to continue doing anything productive during the rest of the day.

On the other hand, powering through that heavy wave of midday drowsiness didn't allow me to work and focus with the same rhythm, either. Long stretches of ceaseless grinding often amounted to very little. That's when I discovered power naps. The nowadays famous power nap is a term that first appeared in the 1998 book titled *Power Sleep* by Dr. James B. Maas, who explained that power naps should consist of phase two non-REM sleep. As explained previously, during this phase, your heart rate and breathing slow down, your body temperature drops, and you start being less aware of your surroundings.

For someone who hasn't tried it yet, dozing off for a few minutes in the middle of the day might not sound that helpful at first; but it turns out that it can indeed have a positive effect on mental clarity, productivity, and recharging when done right.

Boosting Your 7 A.M. Workout Edge with Power Naps

Power naps used to be one of my favorite and most essential productivity tools in the past. Something interesting happened to me, though, once I learned to fine-tune my 7 A.M. Workout Edge. And although I didn't even notice it in the beginning, I one day realized that I hadn't taken a power nap in months! The reason I didn't even realize this for so long was that I wouldn't experience a significant dip in energy or productivity anymore—even when working for ten hours straight! I found that as long as I'm getting enough sleep and sticking to my morning routine, that midday energy dip will either be completely absent or too insignificant to affect me.

I still consider power naps a handy tool, but they're not something I feel I need on a daily basis. They are more of a backup plan to help me get back on track during those weeks when I'm dealing with extra stress or workload, and my sleep is bad or not enough.

Besides these occasions, power naps can also be helpful when you're at the beginning of setting up your morning workout edge. Since you might be still experiencing that midday energy dip at first, power naps can help you to keep going with that little extra boost of energy until you fine-tune everything during the first month and a half!

So, in case you're not familiar with power naps, here is what you need to know when it comes to combining them with the 7 A.M. Workout Edge.

TIP #1: POWER NAPPING IS NOT FOR EVERYONE

Although power naps can be helpful when you're first setting up your morning workout edge, the opposite can be also true! If you're struggling to fall asleep early enough in the evening, or if getting quality deep sleep at night was never your strong point, then I'd then hold off on power naps, especially during the first six weeks of setting up your morning workout edge.

TIP #2: DURATION IS THE KEY

The key to successful power napping is duration. If you fall into deep sleep during your power nap, you'll wake up tired and groggy—the opposite of what a power nap is supposed to do for you. Therefore, your power nap should be long enough to help you feel recharged and continue your day, but not so long that snapping out of it becomes a struggle.

As I've said, maximum recharging during a power nap is achieved by going from stage one sleep (that "drifting off" feeling) to stage two, which is when brain activity starts to slow down. So, how long does that take? I recommend experimenting with anything between fifteen and twenty-five minutes, since this varies from person to person and also from day to day.

For example, on most days, fifteen minutes will do the trick for me. But, if I'm having a day when I'm stressed out, I'll give myself twenty minutes, since I know it will take me a few extra minutes to get comfortable. On these occasions, I'll also start with some mindfulness meditation to allow my racing mind to slow down. This way, if I can't manage to power nap, I at least get a meditation session in. Although, if I compare both in terms of rejuvenation, nothing beats a good power nap!

TIP #3: TIMING IS EVERYTHING

Timing your power nap right is crucial. Most people crash between one and three in the afternoon—usually a little bit after lunch time, since digestion and blood sugar also play a big role in energy regulation. Your wake-up time also affects the time you experience your energy dip, which will usually be about six to eight hours after you get out of bed. So, if you wake up at 6 a.m., your dipping point will probably be somewhere between 12 p.m. and 2 p.m.

Another thing to watch out for is power napping too late. If done after 3 p.m., or six hours or less prior to bedtime, it could have an adverse effect on your night's sleep. Power-napping seven hours prior (or nine hours prior for the more sensitive) to your sleeping time will usually be a safe limit for most people.

TIP #4: SET UP

Finding an appropriate napping spot is crucial! Ideally, this spot should be low-risk in terms of being disturbed by others. If lying down is not an option, the next best option would be a reclining chair. Whatever the case, it's important to find something that allows your back to be reclined and your feet to rest slightly higher than floor level.

Other things I find important are having a quality sleep mask (get a decently soft and comfortable one; it's worth the few extra bucks) and using earplugs, since it's quite bright and noisy at my napping spot. Noise-canceling headphones and nature sounds or white noise can also be helpful for people who power nap in noisy environments.

Whatever your situation is, before you doze off, eliminate as many distractions as possible. Shut the door and put a "Do Not Disturb" sign on it, turn your phone notifications off, and generally do whatever it takes to let people know you are not available for the next half an hour.

P.S. Keep in mind that getting too comfortable might also be a bad idea for those who find it hard to snap out of a power nap. Finding that personal sweet spot that feels *comfortable enough but not too comfortable* is something you want to experiment with.

BONUS TIP: HAVE A NAPPUCCINO

This works great during days when your energy dip is stronger than usual. For me, this is a strategy I'll use on days when I'm severely under-slept and I have a lot on my plate. Nappucinos are a great hack to push through the day on such occasions, and I first heard about them from Daniel Pink, author of *When: The Scientific Secrets of Perfect Timing*.

Having coffee before a nap might sound counterintuitive, but when you keep in mind that it takes about twenty to thirty minutes for caffeine to kick in and start doing its magic, it makes sense. Having a cup of java just before your power nap can help you feel more alert when it's time to snap out of it and avoid that snoozing button.

It helps you avoid sleep-inertia, and it makes it easier to get right back to what it is that you were doing. Specifically, Daniel Pink recommends having a cup of coffee, setting a timer for twenty-five minutes, and kicking back until that timer goes off.

In summary, power naps are proven to improve mood, alertness, and overall health; and they're definitely a much better approach to dealing with your energy dip compared to the typical one of extreme amounts of caffeine or sugar that a lot of people choose. Still, remember that having a power nap that is too long or too late can confuse your body clock and disrupt your sleep during the upcoming night.

Finally, if you suffer from insomnia or have trouble sleeping at night, either skip naps completely or make sure your power naps are done as early in the day as possible, avoiding going over that fifteen to twenty-five minute limit.

CHAPTER 23

ADAPTATIONS & FINE-TUNING

"True refinement seeks simplicity."
—BRUCE LEE

NO MATTER HOW MUCH YOU GET TO ENJOY AND APPRECIATE YOUR MORNING routine and your morning workout edge, periods of staleness are unavoidable. It's just another typical human trait—eventually, there come times during which all our habits feel boring!

Plus, the fact that you came up with what felt like the perfect morning routine at some point doesn't mean that it won't change over time. As you evolve as a person, and as your life changes, your morning routine will have to evolve, as well. Finding ways to keep things fresh is therefore essential. Once again, nothing in this book is set in stone. These are just guidelines to get you started. Later on, after your morning workout routine is established, you can always consider all kinds of personal modifications and fine-tuning.

For example, while trying to finish this book, I started waking up earlier in the morning and squeezing in an hour of writing between my BSR and my morning workout. As I see it, this still doesn't go against any of the main ideas of the book. I still get to train at 7 a.m., which allows me to finish my workout before all the rest of my official adult responsibilities begin.

So, if you feel that your morning routine is becoming rusty, finding ways to freshen it up helps.

Here's what I recommend:

Go through your BSR and the time-tracking challenge from Part 1 and Chapter 1 for a day or two and refine your morning routine once again. Even small adjustments, like changing the type of coffee you drink or listening to a new podcast, can be enough to make things different and get you going again.

Next, if you feel there's something else important you'd like to get done during the peaceful morning hours, you can consider getting up a bit earlier and adding this new habit/task between your BSR and your workout routine. As long as you get enough sleep and you finish your workout before the rest of the day's responsibilities start, you should be fine!

In general, if you want to keep your morning workout edge sharp, it's always a good idea to review and consider refining your morning routine every three to six months! This doesn't mean that you need to make things more complex. Usually, the opposite will be true. The more you keep refining your routine, the more you'll want to seek simplicity.

PART 6

WALK IT OFF

INTRODUCTION

"I said what about my eyes? He said keep them on the road.

"I said what about my passion? He said keep it burning.

"I said what about my heart? He said tell me what you hold inside it?

"I said pain and sorrow. He said stay with it…the wound is the place where the light enters you."
—RUMI

Two things are certain in life…

The first certainty is unpredictability. We never know what is coming our way. Eventually there will be surprises, both good and bad. When I was twenty-three, my life completely changed in the blink of an eye. One moment, I was doing it all—finishing my sports science studies at the university and working two part-time jobs while training for the canoe-kayak national games—and the next moment, I was in a hospital bed wondering if my doctors were going to amputate my leg. If this experience taught me one thing, it's that there is only one antidote for unpredictability: adaptability. As Charles Darwin said: "It's not the strongest of the species that survives, nor the more intelligent. It is the one that is most adaptable to change."

The second certainty is that no one goes through life unwounded. We all end up with scars, some external and plenty internal. Life eventually pierces through our flesh.

It fractures our bones and it breaks our heart, leaving us vulnerable and open. And even though no one is physically or emotionally bulletproof, we do have a choice. We can either detach and become cynical, or we can use our pain and struggles to develop empathy and grow as a person. Having tried both, I can tell you with certainty that the latter works better.

Trying to hide our wounds and withdraw from the world doesn't work. Instead, we must let the light shine through them.

Not Every Morning Will Be Magical

Life can be hard. So hard that it can bring the toughest person to their knees. Eventually, there are phases during which we simply have too many other challenges on our plate to be able to take things such as our morning routine seriously. We can lose our job, our dog can and will die eventually, we can go through a rough divorce, and a loved one can get sick or worse. Sometimes, we might even seem to be struggling without having a clear understanding of what is causing our struggle.

One of the things I've discovered with morning routines is that it's easy to sweep things under the rug of subconsciousness when the world is awake, loud, and busy. But, the morning peace always reflects what is really going on in our psyche. And although I don't want to burst our morning workout edge bubble at this point of the book, I have to mention that not all mornings will be magical and peaceful, even after you reach a point that this seems to be the case more often than not.

So, if after a long period of having experienced all the benefits of the morning workout edge you find yourself going through an inexplicable slump that is more persistent than usual, odds are that there's something else going on. Usually, it's something you're avoiding dealing with.

It's Okay to Hit Pause

In the end, though, you'll see that our morning workout edge routine has its way of keeping us honest with ourselves. It teaches us we can't solve our problems by avoiding them, and that the only way out is through! This means that in order to get over a persistent slump, we have to first identify its root cause, and then take our time to work on it.

Something that is not easy or even common sense, in our age of nonstop busyness mixed with distraction and information overload, is that we sometimes forget how much easier we can make things if we take some time and quiet to focus on actually dealing with our problems instead of waiting for them to magically be solved by themselves.

So, if you're going through a rough patch, it's only normal to hit pause and set your morning workout aside. Falling off the wagon at some point is to be expected, and you shouldn't feel bad about it or force yourself to keep going. Doing this will only lead you to eventually despise your morning routine.

Instead, what's more important during such times is to keep in mind that by having built a habit successfully once, you'll always have the tools to get back at it the moment you feel ready. Sure, you'll experience some resistance in the beginning, but this time, you'll have a head start. You'll see that all it takes to get the ball rolling is following your BSR for a few days, and then the rest will almost effortlessly fall into place!

Until that happens, though, here's what I recommend. If you feel you need some personal time to work on what is burdening you, and yet work and all the rest of your day's responsibilities always seem to suck your mental resources, there's a better way to deal with this as a 7 A.M.-er.

Just walk it off!

CHAPTER 24

WALK IT OFF

"Solvitur ambulando"
—LATIN PHRASE ("IT IS SOLVED BY WALKING")

MORNING WALKS HAVE BEEN THE MOST EFFECTIVE STRATEGY I'VE USED during desperate times to pick myself up again by my own bootstraps. I know walking doesn't sound that powerful, and this would make a very lame fitness influencer post, but my motto is that there aren't a lot of problems a long enough morning walk can't solve!

So, if you're going through a difficult time, for whatever reason, here's what I recommend you do: keep your BSR as it is and replace your morning workout with a plain old simple, good walk.

Walking is one of the physical activities that requires the least amount of motivation, since all you have to do is put one foot in front of the other. Even if you don't feel like doing anything during your morning at this point, walking won't feel as intimidating as working out.

Although exercise in general helps clear the mind, I find that walking is a lot more effective when it comes to using movement to gain insight regarding a problem you're dealing with. Of course, I'm not the first person to say this. It has been acknowledged by everyone from ancient philosophers like Aristotle more than two thousand years ago to people like Zygmunt Freud, from Charles Dickens to Charles Darwin and Winston Churchill, from Apple's Steve Jobs to Facebook's Mark Zuckerberg—who both even did meetings on foot. Many great and successful men and women have talked about the magical problem-solving power of walking.

The way I see it is this: while walking, our mind loosens up and our thoughts come and go in a way that allows us to reorganize them and create the right amount of space between them to spark new, creative connections. This gives different perspectives, and it leads to more original ideas! In other words, walking puts you in a creative-thinking flow-state better than almost anything else!

Although this works any time of the day (which is why I also like to walk in the afternoon as part of my unwinding routine), I've found that the morning peace and clarity provides an even more creatively fertile and contemplative environment to walk in!

By the way, keep in mind that the third golden rule and the general mindset behind our morning routine still applies here. So, don't expect yourself to be able to access that problem-solving walking flow-state with your phone beeping and buzzing in your pocket.

How to Walk It Off

Before I discovered how to apply the problem-solving power of morning walks, I found myself struggling with problems for months when all I had to do was invest a few morning walks into them. Following are some ideas and my personal approach to solving problems with a morning walk. I recommend you give these a try and also create your own strategies.

1. ASK YOURSELF QUESTIONS

Start by observing the most obvious external layers of the problem and asking yourself the most simple questions that pop up in your head. This gives you momentum to start digging deeper.

2. SEARCH FOR THE TRIGGER

Slowly, look for the event that triggered what is causing you unease these days, even if it doesn't seem so significant at a first glance.

3. ADVISE YOURSELF AS IF ADVISING A FRIEND

When it comes to our friends' problems, solutions can be a lot more obvious sometimes. Other than the fact that it's always easier to give advice when you don't have to put in the work, another reason this happens is perspective. Our own problems always come with more emotional charge. We get frustrated and sad, and we can't think in a clear way. However, with other people's problems, we can approach them without getting worked up, and we can perceive them objectively. This allows us to see a lot clearer and give much better advice on how to tackle them.

But you can be your own friend, too. Imagine you are walking with your best friend. Try to tell yourself how you'd get past this obstacle if it were theirs. Focus on the solution and set your emotions aside.

4. TAKE AT LEAST SOME OF THE BLAME

Finally, remember to make sure you take your fair share of blame and don't rush to throw others under the bus first. Most times, even if we're not the root cause of our problems, we do contribute to or prolong them in one way or another. Keep doing this until you have a clear image of your problem.

5. LOOK FOR THE SILVER LINING

Last, but not least, try to look for meaning within your suffering and for the hidden opportunity that may lie within your struggle. As human beings, we are a lot more motivated to change through struggle than we are through comfort. With every big obstacle, there's potential for growth. Ask yourself: how can I evolve through this problem? What are the hidden gains within it? How can I turn this problem into an opportunity to get better, stronger, and tougher?

If you're still stuck, here are some simple questions that I like to ask to stimulate my thinking process:

1. Is there someone or something I am unhappy with right now in my life?

2. If so, what can I do about it? Can I change this person or situation?

3. If not, what can I do on my part to make things easier and cause less discomfort?

4. How can I find meaning within this problem?

5. How can I be more proactive and less reactive?

6. What can I gain from this situation?

7. What's the silver lining behind all this that I might be ignoring?

8. How can I turn all the friction this situation is creating into fuel for positive change?

9. How can I grow as a person from all this experience?

Pick three or four questions to ask yourself per walk, and give the process time. Don't obsess over finding the answers all at once. I find that the more you obsess over the question, the slower the answer appears. It's important to let go and leave some space between asking questions and looking for answers. More often than not, when you let your mind wander off, it comes back with more interesting food for thought (compared to fixating nonstop on the question).

So, in summary, take your problem by the hand each morning and go for a walk with it. Once your morning walk is over, feel free to get busy again with the rest of your day's tasks. Although you won't be aware of it, your mind will keep on working on the problem subconsciously during the rest of the day while you're getting other things done. Sometimes, the answer might even pop out during a random moment of the day as you're doing something completely irrelevant, whether that's in the shower before work, during work, while you're driving back home, or even at the end of the day while having dinner with your family.

Whatever the case, try to keep your attention on other things and revisit your problem consciously the following morning. You'll be surprised, but if you give this a try, you can find answers within a few days to problems you've been looking at for weeks or even months!

The Importance of Talking to a Professional

It goes without saying that if your problem doesn't go away, and you find yourself suffering for too long, it's always a smart idea to talk to a professional. Personally, I'm a big fan of psychotherapy, and after having it done systematically for a year in the past, I can tell you it's one of the best investments I've made in my life. It gave me a huge amount of clarity and helped me evolve as a person, improving my life to a great extent.

CHAPTER 25

FINAL THOUGHTS

"When we are no longer able to change a situation, we are challenged to change ourselves."
—VICTOR FRANKL

THE FIVE YEARS THAT FOLLOWED MY ACCIDENT WERE HARD. I HAD A LOT of rock-bottom moments and frustration that turned into anger that turned into despair. The worst of all, though, is that I wasted a lot of time feeling sorry for myself. After spending most of my twenties in recovery in and out of hospitals and rehabilitation centers, I saw and met plenty of other people dealing with a lot more difficult adversities. In the end, I vowed that once I'd get over my challenge, and as long as I'd be healthy after it, I'd never complain or waste another moment again. I promised myself that after all this, I'd make the best out of my life.

There's a saying that goes as follows: "A sick person has one wish, while a healthy person has a thousand!" I like to paraphrase this quote and say that "a sick person sees one problem, while a healthy person sees a thousand." There will always be periods of struggle, days when we feel down, and times when the world simply doesn't make a lot of sense to us. Even if we don't have a serious reason, it's often human nature to overthink things and to find problems where there are none. No matter how self-actualized we become, it's unavoidable to have our mind slip occasionally and get impatient with goals and wants, to neglect people and situations for which we should be grateful, and, in general, to focus on the negativity around us.

I don't know about you, but I feel that getting side-tracked this way once in a while is almost necessary in order to remember and re-appreciate what is truly important. After all, if I had figured out a way around all this, I'd be writing a book about enlightenment instead.

Whatever we do, our inner world will always oscillate between peace and turbulence. Even after doing all the hard work we can do to arrive at a place of inner calm, life has its way of presenting new, harder obstacles that will cause frustration and throw us off balance again.

A Sense of Purpose

What does all this have to do with the 7 A.M. Workout Edge? Well, the 7 A.M. Workout Edge is not just a smart and practical way to get and stay in shape. It is a practice that can restore inner peace after a previous bad day and help us start the next one with a positive attitude. It's a practice that can help us appreciate each day and try to make the best out of it.

The 7 A.M. Workout Edge is also about making space for that personal quality time with ourselves before our day begins and allowing us to get in touch with a deeper and more pure part of our soul. Although I've searched for spirituality in all kinds of different ways and places, I find that not a lot of things are more spiritual than a cup of coffee warming up my hands as the first morning light appears in the sky—unwrapping hues of blue and orange while the dawn's first birdsongs begin to drift into my kitchen from a half-opened window. My morning workout routine is something I do to get in touch with my sense of purpose, which is always easier to feel while the sun is rising and the world around me is peaceful.

Lastly, it's also something I do to show my appreciation for having a healthy body that gives me independence and carries me around through life on earth.

The 7 A.M. Workout Edge

No, the 7 A.M. Workout Edge isn't a panacea that can fix all your problems. But if you give it time and follow all the steps in this book, each morning has the potential to add a bit more clarity to life's complexity.

So, treat those first peaceful moments of the day as a gift to yourself, and be open to all the details you can appreciate around you. Next, take advantage of your morning workout edge to enter life's daily arena with that unfair advantage! They say that making your bed in the morning makes you more successful because when you start your day with a win it's easier to keep adding more and even bigger wins to the rest of your day. Well, wait until you start your day with a workout!

Notice how, while others are still struggling to wake up, you are already locked and loaded. While others are hanging on the coffee machine at the office, trying to keep their eyes open, you are already attacking that first presentation, client, or task of the day—full throttle!

You're energized, you're in a good mood, you're clear on your goals, and you emit confidence! At the same time, you're calmer and less neurotic, and you connect easier with people, both in the professional and personal realms. And soon enough, others start to notice, as well. It's your boss seeing something special in you as she begins to consider that promotion you've been struggling to get, or maybe it's that special person you've been wanting to ask on a date.

Even if it was more of a dread at first, as time goes by, getting up in the morning becomes more and more reflexive. Eventually, it turns into a well-orchestrated, frictionless routine that you look forward to. It's your secret pocket of personal time that is never trespassed on by the rest of the world that is still snoozing!

Plus, remember all those qualities required to become a successful morning workout person? They also become qualities that make you successful in all of life's fields. By skipping that snooze button, you train yourself to stop postponing the things that truly matter. When you adopt the chef's mindset, you learn to move with purpose and efficiency. When you learn to use your smartphone as a tool and not an infinity vortex of procrastination, you learn to focus on what matters. And suddenly, time begins to slow down to your pace.

And the great thing about all of this is that you don't necessarily need a hardcore workout to get you there! Even a plain, good old power-walk can do the trick for some people. And hey, if you're the more extreme fitness type of personality, you can even get a light workout in the morning, doing just enough to gain that morning workout edge (like a thirty-minute easy jog or calisthenics session), and also do something more intense on top of that later in the day!

After all, different things work for different people!

Whatever the case, remember to be patient in the beginning when you're building this new habit. Just as you won't get in top shape with a "two-weeks to abs" plan, and you won't learn to play the piano or drums after an intense online ten-lesson class, you also won't build a solid morning routine that has the potential to change your life within a few days.

You have to trust the method in this book and give it at least a month and a half before you start jumping to conclusions. Each morning after those six weeks, people start to discover a new version of themselves: someone who is able to set the shallow wants of the ego aside and get aligned with what's truly important. A version that is also more genuine and worth getting to know better.

I hope you enjoyed this book and, most importantly, that you'll put everything you read into practice.

—Anthony

For all the supplementary materials and extra information mentioned in the book, please visit: www.the7AMworkoutedge.com.

ABOUT THE AUTHOR

MY NAME IS ANTHONY ARVANITAKIS, AND I'M A GRADUATE OF THE SPORTS science and physical education department at the Aristotle University of Thessaloniki. I'm a health and wellness coach and an author of bestselling books on Amazon, such as *Bodyweight Muscle.* Helping people get in their best shape without lifting weights or using fancy machines, aka calisthenics, has been my passion for the last decade.

After an accident in my early twenties that cost me my left leg and left me depressed and in the worst shape of my life, I got obsessed with bodyweight training and managed to turn things around by creating a positive and healthy lifestyle, with calisthenics and morning exercise as two of its main pillars.

Made in United States
North Haven, CT
19 May 2023

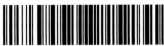

36718683R00152